Making the DSM-5

Joel Paris • James Phillips
Editors

Making the DSM-5

Concepts and Controversies

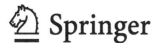 Springer

Editors
Joel Paris, MD
Jewish General Hospital
Department of Psychiatry
McGill University
Montreal, QC, Canada

James Phillips, MD
Department of Psychiatry
Yale School of Medicine
New Haven, CT, USA

ISBN 978-1-4614-6503-4   ISBN 978-1-4614-6504-1 (eBook)
DOI 10.1007/978-1-4614-6504-1
Springer New York Heidelberg Dordrecht London

Library of Congress Control Number: 2013932650

Printed on acid-free paper

Springer is part of Springer Science+Business Media (www.springer.com)

Preface

In 2013, the American Psychiatric Association is publishing the fifth edition of its Diagnostic and Statistical Manual of Mental Disorders (DSM-5). This book examines some of the conceptual and pragmatic issues raised by the new manual.

DSM has sometimes been called "the bible of psychiatry." This seems a strange term to describe a manual that only classifies mental disorders, but does not explain them or guide their treatment. Yet while earlier editions of DSM had little impact on clinical practice, DSM-III, published in 1980, was a kind of "paradigm shift," reflecting the shift of focus in American psychiatry from psychodynamics to phenomenology and neuroscience. Moreover, DSM-III introduced algorithms for diagnosis that proved popular, even if they were not followed very strictly. This edition of the manual became influential all over the world, and also became a standard for almost all research.

The controversy over DSM-III eventually blew over. Biological psychiatry won the day, and was accepted as the primary paradigm for the field. DSM-IV, published in 1994, made only minor changes in the manual. Thirty odd years later, few could remember a psychiatry that did not follow the DSM. However flawed the system was, the pace of research was slow, and most mental disorders remained poorly understood.

Nonetheless, the American Psychiatric Association felt it was time for a revision. To this end, they appointed David Kupfer, a prominent biological researcher, and Darryl Regier, their own research director, to head a task force to prepare DSM-5. This process took quite a few years, with work groups of experts asked to propose revisions based on the most recent research findings. Originally, APA hoped to introduce another paradigm shift, in which psychiatric diagnosis would be in greater harmony with neuroscience. When it became clear the data supporting these changes was too fragmentary for radical changes, it backed off from major revisions.

The final document that constitutes DSM-5 is a compromise. It is not dramatically different from DSM-IV, but reflects a tendency to see mental disorders as lying on a continuum with normality, and supports the view that half of the population can be labeled as having some kind of mental disorder. It is hoped that this model will eventually be supported by the discovery of biological markers and endophenotypes.

The chapters in this book examine DSM-5 from the point of view of these conceptual principles, and also assess the implications of its approach for clinical practice.

Several chapters consider the problem of over-diagnosis and false positives. Psychiatry has long been criticized for medicalizing and pathologizing normal variations, and over-diagnosis means over-treatment, with all the attendant side-effects of psychopharmacological interventions. At the same time, some conditions listed in DSM-5 may be underdiagnosed. This "dialectic" can best be resolved by a combination of conservatism and pragmatism. Diagnostic epidemics could discredit psychiatry by claiming that there is no essential difference between mental disorder and normality, and by forcing clinicians to treat normal people with drugs that they do not need.

One must also consider the political and economic context in which over-diagnosis occurs. The history and politics of American psychiatry is marked by a need to stand equal to other medical specialties. The creation of the new manual is seen as an attempt to create a system that is consistent with neuroscience, but that goes beyond existing data. At the same time, psychiatry hopes to legitimate itself with a scientific diagnostic system. But in DSM-5, the overall definition of mental disorder in the manual is weak, failing to distinguish psychopathology from normality. Moreover, there are powerful interests, both corporate and, public, that could profit from a highly inclusive diagnostic system.

Finally, we have to address the question of whether the vision of psychiatry guiding DSM-5 is valid. Its scientific theory corresponds to a medical approach, but does not distinguish "disease" from "illness." Thus diagnoses in psychiatry may not be "natural kinds." DSM-5 raises both conceptual and pragmatic problems that will affect the future of psychiatry. In the years to come, it will be subjected to detailed empirical testing. At the same time, the diagnostic system needs to adopt a broader model that does not reduce all of psychopathology to neuroscience. These developments could eventually lead to a better system for DSM-6.

Montreal, QC, Canada   Joel Paris

Contents

Contributors

Allen Frances Department of Psychiatry, Duke University, Durham, NC, USA

Allan V. Horwitz Department of Sociology and Institute for Health, Health Care Policy, and Aging Research, Rutgers University, New Brunswick, NJ, USA

Warren Kinghorn Department of Psychiatry and Behavioral Sciences, Duke University Medical Center and Duke Divinity School, Durham, NC, USA

Aaron L. Mishara Department of Clinical Psychology, Sofia University, Palo Alto, CA, USA

Joel Paris Jewish General Hospital, Department of Psychiatry, McGill University, Montreal, QC, Canada

James Phillips Department of Psychiatry, Yale School of Medicine, New Haven, CT, USA

Joseph M. Pierre Department of Psychiatry and Biobehavioral Sciences, David Geffen School of Medicine at UCLA, Los Angeles, CA, USA

VA Greater Los Angeles Healthcare System, Los Angeles, CA, USA

Douglas Porter Central City Behavioral Health Center, New Orleans, LA, USA

John Z. Sadler Department of Psychiatry, The University of Texas, Southwestern Medical Center, Dallas, TX, USA

Michael A. Schwartz Departments of Psychiatry and Humanities in Medicine Texas A & M Health Science Center College of Medicine, Round Rock, TX, USA

Edward Shorter Faculty of Medicine, University of Toronto, ON, Canada

Owen Whooley Department of Sociology, University of New Mexico, Albuquerque, NM, USA

Part I
Historical/Ideological Perspectives

Chapter 1
The History of DSM

Edward Shorter

> *At Ohio's Academy GP meeting one year, I gave a paper on the [new] drugs, and in the discussion afterwards, a man got up and said: 'Very erudite paper, but it isn't worth a damn to me, because when you say don't give this drug to an obsessive compulsive, this drug is good in an endogenous depression, you are talking way over my head. The doctor sitting next to me might be schizophrenic or he may have an endogenous depression, I wouldn't know this.'*
>
> —Frank Ayd, one of the pioneering psychopharmacologists, at the founding meeting of the American College of Neuropsychopharmacology, 1960 [1].

Psychiatric diagnosis turns out to be complicated, probably far more so than anyone thought 50 years ago in the heyday of psychoanalysis when diagnosis didn't really count. And the story of the Diagnostic and Statistical Manual of the American Psychiatric Association is, at one level, a tale of steady progress in getting things right. At another level, it is the story of a nosological process that has, to some extent, run off the rails. Despite enormous investments of time, thought, and academic firepower, the means of establishing a reliable nosology of psychiatric illness continues to slip from our grasp.

Psychiatry has always had a nosology, or roster of classifying diseases according to some basic principle. The motto of no treatment without diagnosis is as valid in psychiatry as in any other specialty. And modern systems of classification, detached from the humoralism of the Ancients, go back to such seminal writers as Philippe Pinel in Paris [2] and August Heinroth in Leipzig [3]. Yet how reluctant nature has

E. Shorter (✉)
Faculty of Medicine, University of Toronto, 150 College St, #83D, Toronto, ON M5S 3E2, Canada
e-mail: edwardshorter@gmail.com

J. Paris and J. Phillips (eds.), *Making the DSM-5: Concepts and Controversies*, DOI 10.1007/978-1-4614-6504-1_1, © Springer Science+Business Media New York 2013

been to give up her secrets! In presenting the new diagnosis delirious mania—later seen as a form of malignant catatonia—to the profession in 1849, Luther V Bell, chief physician at the McLean Asylum for the Insane in a suburb of Boston, lamented the difficulty of digging a new disease entity "from the mass of rubbish— of confused, irregular conglomerations of amorphous appearance, to separate it from the encumbrance of incidental matters, and so present it, that others may be able to satisfy themselves of its genuine individuality" [4].

Anticipating DSM

As medicine established itself increasingly as a science rather than an art in the course of the nineteenth century, the demand became loud within psychiatry for a system of classification that went beyond the rough categories of Pinel and Heinroth. In 1851 Louis Delasiauve, a veteran psychiatrist at Bicêtre mental hospital in Paris, scorned his colleagues for their uninterest in diagnosis, leading to anarchy in treatment. "I have been preoccupied over almost the entire course of my career with ways of putting an end to this. And it seems to me that the comparative study of different kinds of types, and of the analogies they have in common as well as the differences that separate them, is calculated to lead to more satisfactory data on which a nomenclature might be based" [5]. But how to derive such data?

There are three approaches to creating a nosology: reliance on authority, on consensus, or, the third, by identifying a disease by the "medical model," a well-defined process that depends on more than "consensus" in opinion or symptoms alone. At the origins of twentieth-century classifications of psychiatric illness was the principle of authority, namely the authority of Emil Kraepelin, the great German nosologist who taught in Heidelberg and in Munich. Kraepelin simply sat in the quiet of his study, deliberated, then communicated to the profession his views about disease classifications, which thereupon were almost universally adopted. (He was, of course, a very active clinician as well.) This process began with the first edition of Kraepelin's textbook in 1883 [6] and reached its maximum influence with the massive eighth edition, the last one he was to create himself [7]. The innovative aspect of the Kraepelinian system was its intention of predicting prognosis. Not the phenomenology as such determined illness classification, but "how things are going to progress," as Kraepelin's colleague Robert Gaupp put it in 1926, the year Kraepelin died. "The prognosis is the touchstone of all of our science" [8]. In an epoch that lacked effective treatments, the ability to foretell a patient's future was the very rationale of nosology.

With the sixth edition in 1899, Kraepelin made several distinctions that are still with us. He had already originated in earlier editions the diagnosis dementia praecox, which became schizophrenia in 1908 under Eugen Bleuler's pen [9]. But in 1899 Kraepelin erected a firewall between the psychosis of dementia praecox and the affective troubles of manic-depressive illness [10]. Thus the two great illnesses of psychiatry became schizophrenia and "MDI," as different from each other as chalk and cheese and, for the most part, never destined to meet, or converge.

Yet authoritarian as he was in imposing his own concepts, in a sense, on the entire world, Kraepelin was also quite thoughtful about the requirements of successful nosology: the purpose was, as he explained in 1894, to create small, homogeneous groups of patients whose illnesses had "the same etiology, course, duration, and outcome." (He gave the presentation verbally in 1892 at a psychiatric meeting but the abstract was published only in 1894 [11].) Indeed, this is the holy grail of nosology, with differential responsiveness to medication added in today.

At an international level, the tradition of determining nosology by eminent experts rather than committees continued with Aubrey Lewis, professor of psychiatry at the Maudsley Hospital after the Second World War. Lewis angled towards the view that it was not useful to distinguish between "endogenous" and "exogenous" forms of depressive illness [12]. Yet Lewis never wrote a textbook and failed to have the same comprehensive impact on nosology that Kraepelin did. In these years the continent fell silent as a source of innovative thought because of war and the Holocaust (with a few exceptions [13]), and the baton passed across the ocean to the United States and the DSM series of the American Psychiatric Association.

The DSM series began with a document much in the tradition of authoritarian pronunciamentos rather than consensus. On October 19, 1945, psychoanalyst William Menninger, in charge of psychiatric services for the US Army during World War II, promulgated on his own a diagnostic roster, called Technical Medical Bulletin no. 203, which became the immediate ancestor of the DSM series [14]. (One recalls that in these years Army psychiatry was permeated with psychoanalysis. Max Fink describes attending the Army School of Military Neuropsychiatry at Fort Sam Houston in 1946, where the curriculum was one third general psychiatry, one third neurology, and one third psychoanalysis [15].) "Medical 203," as Menninger's creation came to be called, bore an immediate Freudian flavor, dwelling at length upon "psychoneurotic disorders... resulting from the exclusion from the consciousness (i.e., repression) of powerful emotional charges, usually attached to certain infantile and childhood developmental experiences." Chief of these disorders was "anxiety," always the vaulting stone of the Freudian edifice. Menninger spoke of "anxiety reactions... unconsciously and automatically controlled by the utilization of various psychological defense mechanisms (repression, conversion, displacement, etc.)" [14].

Yet Medical 203 also bore the Kraepelinian imprint that would spill over 7 years later into the DSM series. "Psychotic disorders," meaning serious illness, constituted a separate category. And they were separated into watertight compartments: First were "schizophrenic disorders," also called, in the tradition of Adolf Meyer at Johns Hopkins University, "reactions." Kraepelin's three schizophrenic subtypes— hebephrenic, catatonic, and paranoid—were in attendance, and chronic "paranoia," without deterioration of the personality, was, as in the Kraepelinian system, singled out as separate. Then came "affective disorders," led by "manic-depressive reaction" and quite distinct from schizophrenia. This was the firewall.

Menninger distinguished among manic-depressive illness, psychotic depression, and Kraepelin's involutional melancholia. (Curious that Menninger should have retained involutional melancholia, the serious depression of midlife, after Kraepelin himself had rejected the diagnosis and made it part of MDI.) All these nosological decisions would shortly reappear in DSM-I.

DSM-I and DSM-II

In 1951 the US Public Health Service organized a working party under George Raines, who was the representative of the American Psychiatric Association, to consider revising the sixth edition of World Health Organization's International Classification of Diseases (ICD-6) [16] to bring it into correspondence with American usage. It was the output of that group that eventuated in 1952 in the first edition of the DSM series, later known as "DSM-I." Led by Raines, 44 in 1952, a former Navy neuropsychiatrist and then professor of psychiatry at Georgetown University Medical Center, DSM-I hewed fairly closely to Medical 203. It was, of course much longer and more comprehensive, yet the same psychoneuroses were laid out in detail, as were the same psychoses, which included manic-depressive illness (in the Kraepelinian sense, meaning mania and all forms of depression except neurotic depression) and schizophrenia. Medical 203 had spoken of psychotic disorders "without known organic etiology." DSM-I attributed these psychoses to "disturbance of metabolism, growth, nutrition or endocrine function" [17]. The main intellectual differences between the two documents were actually trivial, and DSM-I carried on the Meyerian tradition of labeling psychiatric disorders "reactions." Interestingly, of the six other members of the drafting committee, only one—Moses Frohlich—was an analyst, and several others had backgrounds that were military or in neuropsychiatry, or were colleagues at Georgetown.

DSM-I was virtually without influence on the international scene, although by 1967 it had reached 20 printings in the United States. Yet, with the possible exception of the WHO's own classification, promulgated in 1957, none of the other nosologies current at the time had been influential either [13]. It was the explosion of new psychopharmacologic agents in the 1950s that made the field sit up and take notice of nosology. Yet this did not have an undilutedly favorable influence on psychiatry's ability to make the kind of fine diagnostic differentiations that nosology calls for, which entails a sense of differential responsiveness.

What are the diagnoses that respond differentially to different agents? The conventional assumption was that the new drugs encouraged diagnostic differentiation, because it made a difference in prescribing whether your patient had an affective illness or schizophrenia. This may have applied in combatting the influence of psychoanalysis in the United States, where the new drugs reinforced the firewall between manic-depression and psychosis. In the US Max Fink and Donald Klein used the new drugs as a kind of "pharmacological torch" for distinguishing one disease from another [18]. But in Europe the new psychopharmacology, if anything, discouraged old traditions of fine psychopathologic differentiation. The Germans once made elaborate refinements among the different kinds of psychotic illness, and Christian Müller's Psychiatric Dictionary goes on for nine pages about the different courses of the variant forms of psychosis [19]. Yet with the new antipsychotic medications none of this differentiation mattered: all forms responded equally to chlorpromazine. As pioneering French psychopharmacologist Pierre Lambert lamented to the Collegium Internationale Neuro-Psychopharmacologicum (CINP) at its founding meeting in Rome in 1958, "The classification of the patients, and their assignment to a more elaborated clinical entity according to a minute description of their symptoms, is a task that has been practically abandoned," an unfortunate consequence, he said, of the new psychopharmacology and loss of interest in "psychiatric nosology" [20]. So in at least part of the Atlantic community, the most thrilling development in psychiatry for years—the eruption of successful drug treatments—was working not in favor of sophisticated nosology but against it.

Meanwhile, in the United States the APA published DSM-II in 1968. It was, again, a desire to bring US nosology into accordance with the WHO's ICD series (this time ICD-8) that gave rise to DSM-II, and throughout the 1960s several international committees coordinated the drafting of the two documents [21]. (Why the United States wanted its own classification, that eventuated in ICD-9-CM in 1978, is an interesting question: the APA seems to have clung to psychoanalysis and feared the Europeans would impose concepts alien to the US psychiatric culture.)

Unlike its predecessor, DSM-II featured psychoanalysis on the bowsprit. Jointly led by Ernest Gruenberg, a Columbia professor who was not a psychoanalyst, and analyst Lawrence C. Kolb, director of the New York State Psychiatric Institute, the five other members of the committee included only one further analyst, Henriette Klein. But the document had a Freudian ring.

The meat and drink were the sections on "psychoses" and what had been called "psychoneurotic disorders" but that by 1968 had become "neuroses." "Schizophrenic reactions" had become in DSM-II "schizophrenia," a single disease (and, in psychoanalysis, little more than a defense against anxiety). Reactions in general were gone, and among the new neuroses introduced in 1968 was the classic psychoanalytic chestnut "hysterical neurosis." (The 1952 Manual had known only "conversion reaction" and "dissociative reaction.") What was hysterical neurosis? "An involuntary psychogenic loss or disorder of function. Symptoms characteristically begin and end suddenly in emotionally charged situations and are symbolic of the underlying conflicts" [21]. Neurasthenia, also once a favorite of Freud's, had been revived as "neurasthenic neurosis." Commented Henry Davidson, superintendent of a psychiatric hospital in New Jersey, "If we are going to take hysteria out of storage, polish it up and reinstate it, why then 'hysterical neurosis?' Why not just plain hysteria?" As well, "The dreadfully outmoded word 'neurasthenia' is back at the old stand. We are really better off without it. It is too easy a waste-basket for almost anything we can't explain and it has a wretchedly 1910 flavor about it. Better let it go with the horse-cars" (Davidson HA to Gruenberg EM, 1967 Mar 30; APA Archives (Arlington VA), Medical Director's Office, Range 37, box E-2, DSM II: "Comments on the new nomenclature.")

To recap: In the early DSMs, depression had been handled in two ways:

1. Kraepelin's manic-depressive illness had been considered a major affective disorder, part of the "psychoses" that also included schizophrenia; this meant that depression of both polarities, bipolar and melancholic unipolar, were lumped together.
2. Neurotic depression was part of the "neuroses," along with phobic neurosis, obsessive-compulsive neurosis, and so forth.

This division was much in keeping with the traditional psychiatric view that there were two very different depressions, different diseases really, the one melancholic, the other nonmelancholic, or neurasthenic, reactive, neurotic, characterological, or whatever was the adjective of the day.

A young biometrician at the New York State Psychiatric Institute named Robert Spitzer had been named "consultant" to DSM-II. He couldn't wait to get rid of hysteria, neurasthenia, and the rest of the psychoanalytic baggage. He would shortly have his chance.

DSM-III

After DSM-II, psychiatric diagnosis in the United States began to seem increasingly unsatisfactory. For one thing, the diagnosis "schizophrenia" was vastly overused, manic-depressive illness by contrast much ignored [22]. This was because the analysts had a tropism towards what they called schizophrenia as something they could work with. As Jerome Frank at Johns Hopkins University explained at a meeting of the American Psychopathological Association in 1971 (published in 1972), "The depressed patient is a poor candidate for psychotherapy. He interacts sparsely with others, is dull and unproductive, sees the world in an impoverished and stereotyped way, and really wants to be left alone." As well, said Frank, the depressed patient responded readily to such non-psychotherapeutic treatments as electroshock and antidepressants. "Young schizophrenics, on the other hand, are considered in the United States to be ideal candidates for psychotherapy—at least, psychotherapy with them is always a rewarding and challenging experience for the therapist. They have a rich inner life, are very sensitive to nuances in interpersonal behavior, and the therapeutic relationship is a lively and eventful one with constant shifts and challenges" [23]. Yet this happy state of affairs gave American diagnosis a peculiar cast in international perspective and was unacceptable in a discipline with increasingly scientific pretensions.

The powder train that led to DSM-III in 1980 began in April 1969 when Martin Katz, chief of the clinical research branch in the extramural program of the National Institute of Mental Health (NIMH), convened in Williamsburg, Virginia, a conference on "the psychobiology of the depressive illnesses." After decades of psychoanalysis, it was finally time to hear about depression and biology, and a who's who of big names in the biological side of the field, among them Eli Robins, head of psychiatry at the country's premier biological department, Washington University in St Louis, came together at the College of William and Mary to talk about such issues as "electrolyte changes in the affective disorders" [24]. At the meeting the idea germinated that it was time to take a closer look at the classification of psychiatric illness in light of the new biological learning. This was also the beginning of NIMH's major "Collaborative Study" in the biology of depression, which in the view of psychiatric epidemiologist Myrna Weissman "brought depression to the forefront" [25].

In 1972 the first step on the road to DSM-III was trod when the Washington University group, led by Eli Robins and Samuel Guze, proposed an innovative new nosology that would be guided by such Wash U principles as careful description, verification, and validation. It was mainly the doing of the residents, inspired by the teachings of Guze and Robins, who met in Robins's office every Wednesday for months, as Paula Clayton, then a resident herself though not involved in these discussions, remembers it [26]. Robins himself was increasingly ill. Senior resident John Feighner took the initiative of writing up the diagnoses. Fritz Henn, also a resident at the time, later said, "We all sat around a table and simply made these criteria up from the old Kraepelin stuff. The idea was to be able to communicate with each other and form homogeneous groups" [27]. The residents' work—together with input from department members—appeared in 1972 as the "Washington University diagnostic criteria."

The Feighner group boiled down diagnoses quite radically. Gone were Kraepelin's manic-depressive illness and the psychoanalysts' neurotic depression. In their place arose simply "primary affective disorders: depression." Mania was another primary affective disorder. Then came schizophrenia and four of Freud's neuroses, and that was it for the main psychiatric diagnoses.

Highly innovative was the introduction of operational criteria required to get a patient into any particular diagnosis. For depression, for example, were required dysphoric mood plus at least five of eight specific criteria (e.g., loss of energy, sleep difficulty), plus an illness duration of at least a month and not caused by some other preexisting psychiatric condition [28]. This kind of fine attention to symptoms was a radical break with the psychoanalytic tradition of uninterest in symptoms and concentration on supposed intrapsychic conflict.

Shortly after the appearance of Feighner's diagnostic criteria, Martin Katz contacted Endicott, Spitzer, and Robins to create the Research Diagnostic Criteria (RDC) [29]. Spitzer and Endicott were at the New York State Psychiatric Institute, often called "PI." Spitzer, 40 years old in 1972, had trained in psychiatry at PI and was a member of the biometrics unit under Joseph Zubin. His contact with clinical psychiatry had been minimal. But he was a veritable font of enthusiasm and charismatic charm, and if anyone were equipped to overturn the massive psychoanalytic enterprise, it would be he. Endicott, 36, was a psychologist at PI and contributed sound common sense throughout the entire exercise. Spitzer and Endicott made several trips to St. Louis, staying at Robins's, and a collaborative effort began to evolve between the two groups.

These efforts reached initial fruition in 1975 with the RDC being tried on psychiatric case records. Authored principally by Spitzer, Endicott, and Robins, the RDC introduced the fateful distinction into American psychiatry between "bipolar disorder" and unipolar depression, which latter the RDC divided into "major depressive disorder" and "minor depressive disorder." Given that bipolar disorder (as distinct from unipolar depression) had originated in 1957 from German nosologist Karl Leonard, its American beachhead was led by the Wash U group, especially Winokur and Clayton [30]. But the major depression concept was refined into ten subtypes [31]. And minor depression included anxiety, giving American psychiatry definitively a mixed depression-anxiety conception to take the place of "nervous disease" of yore [32]. The definitive version of RDC published in 1978 was essentially the nosology of 1975, with the addition of splitting bipolar disorder into types I (with mania) and II (with hypomania), but this would shortly vanish [33]. In a way, with its many finely differentiated diagnoses, the RDC represented the apex of postwar American nosology; so much of this was to disappear from DSM-III, a testimonial to the political pressure Spitzer was under in dealing with the American Psychiatric Association but freed from in RDC.

But let's not get ahead of our story. In 1974, keen to keep American diagnostics in step with the new draft of the World Health Organization's ever evolving ICD series, the APA appointed Spitzer head of a task force to rejig American psychiatric nosology. Why Spitzer, a relatively junior and unknown figure? Donald Klein later said, "Bob Spitzer got the job after they offered it to Henry Brill [former deputy commissioner of the New York State Department of Mental Hygiene], who turned it down, saying he wasn't interested. Spitzer got the job because it was unimportant. The whole notion of diagnosis was just a nuisance and not really central to anybody's concern" [34].

The APA leadership had no idea what they had let themselves in for. Spitzer intended a fundamental re-creation of psychiatry's diagnoses. In keeping with the emerging alliance between Washington University and the New York State Psychiatric Institute, Spitzer appointed a Task Force with heavy representations from both camps: Robert Woodruff, Donald Goodwin, and Nancy Andreasen from the Wash U camp, and then Paula Clayton after Woodruff committed suicide. From PI came Donald Klein, who along with Max Fink was then the single most powerful voice in American nosology, Rachel Gittelman, who was married to Klein, and Endicott. Interestingly, at heated moments in the discussion, key corridor decisions were made by PI staffers such as Edward Sachar, the director, who were not even members of the Task Force! Although several members, including Spitzer and Don Klein, had been trained as analysts, by 1968 they had turned their backs on Freud and were reaching out to the new biology.

In the background of these events were Spitzer's boss Joe Zubin, and Gerald Klerman, who might be considered the fixer of American psychiatry. In 1980 52 years old and professor of psychiatry at Harvard, Klerman's fingerprint appears nowhere on the printed text yet his views were given great weight, and some feel that DSM basically gave up on classifying depressions after Klerman made it seem of such complexity [35]. As Thomas Ban observes, "It is true that Bob Spitzer did much of the work, but it was really Zubin and in some way Klerman who were trying to pursue the line that began with Kraepelin using his Zählkarten [one-page case summaries], in developing a diagnostic classification in mental illness by using psychometrics. If the DSM-III people had pursued it clean without mixing it with a consensus-based approach for identifying syndromes, they would have created something to build on" (Ban TA, personal communication, 2012 Jul 15).

In September 1974 as the Task Force was getting organized, a number of key decisions were made (Task Force on Nomenclature and Statistics, 1974 Sep 4–5; APA Archives, Professional Affairs, box 17, folder 188). First of all, so much for the proposed revision of ICD. Spitzer said, "We should decide what the new nomenclature should be, then see how it fits with ICD-9, rather than try to prepare a new nomenclature to be congruent with ICD-9." How about the specific diagnoses? "They may reflect etiology," said Spitzer, thus completely negating the later mantra of DSM-III, issued to counter the psychoanalysts, that DSM was a neutral with respect to etiology. "Functional" was deemed no longer suitable as a classification of disorders, "which are no longer seen as purely psychogenic." The distinction between "psychosis" and "neurosis" was also considered useless. A number of important decisions seem to have been taken by Spitzer alone. In drawing up the advisory committees on the individual diagnostic basins he quite arbitrarily decided to make the committee that would consider depression separate from the committee that dealt with anxiety. This virtually guaranteed that mixed anxiety-depression, the previous workhorse of non-psychoanalytic psychiatry, would vanish from the stage. But this was a detail. For the members of the Task Force, in September 1974, it was a new dawn.

Yet once the disease-designers were at the negotiating table, their approach more resembled horse-trading than admiration for science. Take "schizophrenia," which emerged from the published DSM-III as seemingly rock-solid a diagnosis as mumps. As psychologist Theodore Millon, member of the DSM-III Task Force, pointed out to Spitzer in 1978, this label—for what is essentially chronic psychosis— had begun life in DSM-I as "schizophrenic reaction" and was simplified to "schizophrenia" in DSM-II in 1968. Then, as the DSM-III Task Force began to meet, they converted it in 1974 into "schizophrenic disorders" in recognition, said Millon, that the term represented "a spectrum, if you will, that is, a heterogeneous syndrome, etiologically biogenic in some cases, psychogenic in others, and most likely interactive in the majority." Then, to Millon's irritation, in 1978 Spitzer unilaterally reconverted the label to "schizophrenia," as it remained in the published version (Millon T, memo to Task Force Members, 1978 Jul 16; ACNP-ULCA Archive (Los Angeles, CA), Paula Clayton papers, box 30, folder 15). So, schizophrenia, was it one disease or a haphazard catchall? The DSM system was all over the map.

Secondly, the horse-trading with the psychoanalysts of the contents of DSM-III resulted in several distortions. From the outset, the analysts hated the draft DSM's proposed exclusion of the term "neurosis" and the rejection of "intrapsychic conflict" as the motor of mental distress. In January 1979 Marilyn Skinner, a New Orleans analyst and chairperson of the APA's oversight committee of the Task Force, complained of DSM-III's efforts "to classify descriptively rather than dynamically." The Task Force had split up the neuroses into "several categories," she said, "affective, anxiety, somatoform, and dissociative disorders." She was especially unhappy about "the inclusion of the (formerly) neurotic depression under affective disorders. This is a blatant instance of an implied disregard for psychodynamic factors" (Skinner M, memo to Jensen M, 1979 Jan 15; APA Archives, Records of the Assembly, box 19, folder 275). This note was typical of a tidal wave of protest from the analysts that bore down on Spitzer, forcing him to act in order to get the document through the APA's Assembly. So Spitzer restored "neurosis."

Thus, in April 1979 "dysthymic disorder," a concept that had been circling in discussion, became suddenly concrete (Spitzer, letter to Task Force, 1979 Apr 30; APA Archives, Janet BW Williams papers, DSM-III-R, loose DSM-III files. "Neurosis" folder); and in the published DSM dysthymia was described in parentheses as "depressive neurosis."

Donald Klein's reply to Spitzer about this decision was scorching and got to the heart of the whole problem with DSM-III: "I must admit that I was flabbergasted by this memo." He scored Spitzer's authoritarian, unilateral decision. "Your current stand is, as far as I can see, entirely your own creation and was taken without either consultation with the Task Force or its agreement" (Klein to Spitzer, Your Memorandum of 3/27/79 and "possible neurotic peace treaty" procedural issues, 1979 Mar 30; ACNP-UCLA Archive, Clayton papers, box 31). In a second memo to the Task Force, also written that day, Klein added that Spitzer's insertion of neurosis into their work "is clearly a response to political pressure, rather than a conceptual advance... To respond to this sort of unscientific and illogical, but sociologically understandable, pressure in the fashion that Dr. Spitzer suggests is unworthy of scientists who are attempting to advance our field via clarification and reliable definition" (Klein, Memo to Members of the DSM-III task force & consultants. Substantive review of memo of March 27, 1979, of Dr. Spitzer in reference: neurotic peace treaty. 1979 Mar 30; ACNP-UCLA Archive, Clayton papers, box 31). This of course was the nub: DSM-III was a political, not a scientific document.

And here is the problem as we try to assess the DSM series within the force field of eminent-authority vs. committee-consensus nosology. On the face of it, the committee ruled, and the DSM-III drafters held many votes about which scientific issue was correct. Yet above these squabbling committees and their compromises lurked Spitzer—if the metaphor is pardonable—as a kind of master puppeteer, who invariably arranged for the outcome that he personally wished. Why were biological markers never considered in the DSM criteria? Spitzer later said, in an interview, that the subject simply never came up on the Task Force (Spitzer R, interview with Shorter E and Fink M, 2007 Mar 14). Yet in 1981 we find Task Force member Paula Clayton advocating the dexamethasone suppression test in differentiating depression from dementia [36]. She must have spoken up on the Task Force, or was her voice simply overruled?

Consequences of DSM-III

In retrospect, DSM-III was a historic document because it rescued American psychiatry from psychoanalysis, marking the beginning of the end of Freud's influence. This was not lost on the analysts, who saw big, unhappy changes coming. As Boyd Burris, president of the Baltimore-District of Columbia Society for Psychoanalysis, wrote to fellow analyst Jules Masserman, then president of the APA, in April 1979, "Unfortunately for us, DSM-III in its present version would seem to have all the earmarks for causing an upheaval in American psychiatry which will not soon be put down" (Burris to Masserman J, 1979 Apr 18; ACNP-UCLA Archive, Clayton papers, box 31).

In terms of diagnoses, DSM-III continued the concrete nosology of the St. Louis School, which, turning diagnoses into diseases, was intended to put maximum daylight between American psychiatry and psychoanalysis. Major depression, infantile autism, schizotypal personality disorder (laid out in RDC), and attention deficit disorder were among the big new diagnoses. Bipolar disorder, as we have seen, was introduced in RDC but had not been in DSM-II. On and on went the list: foreshadowed by RDC, anxiety neurosis had dissolved into panic disorder and generalized anxiety disorder. New was that drug dependence had given way to substance use. The innovations and neologisms were many. Psychiatric theorist David Healy later said that this was the big story in American psychiatry yet the media had missed it: "The neuroses have been medicalized. Panic disorder, OCD and now social phobia have been made disease entities. It has all happened seemingly without the media being aware about what has happened" [37].

Nor were the media aware that DSM-III had introduced several highly problematical diagnoses into world psychiatry:

1. "Schizophrenia" as a single disease
2. "Major depression" as a single clinical entity, instead of keeping psychiatry's previous two depressions separate
3. "Bipolar disorder" as distinct from unipolar depression; many authorities believe that bipolar disorder is nothing more than melancholic depression complicated with the occasional eruption of mania, which is standard in melancholic illness [38]

DSM-III also abolished "mixed anxiety depression" of the RDC, a disease entity that, along with neurotic depression, had been the commonest form of depressive illness in American psychiatry in the first half of the twentieth century [32]. All of a sudden—poof!—it was gone. These issues would complicate diagnosis and treatment for decades to come.

The new nosology also complicated things for the pharmaceutical industry. On the one hand, the DSM-III diagnoses were a gift, handing industry "diseases" on a plate for which they could indicate agents that previously had only such vague labels as "anxiety." On the other hand, the FDA would insist henceforth that industry use DSM-III diagnoses in drug development. As Paul Leber, head of neuropharmacology at FDA said in November, 1980, "The diagnostic system of choice is DSM-III. You may use another one. However, a DSM-III classification of every patient is required" (US Food and Drug Administration (Silver Spring, MD), Psychopharmacologic Drugs Advisory Committee, 18th meeting, 1980 Nov 6, p. 162; obtained through the Freedom of Information Act). This was a Danaean gift, a poisoned chalice, as industry would soon learn in trying to discover and develop drugs for such heterogeneous indications as "major depression."

DSM-III changed psychiatric diagnosis. Paul McHugh and Phillip Slavney at Johns Hopkins University later said that diagnosis had altered from a bottom-up process to top-down. Previously, bottom-up diagnosis was "based on a detailed life history, painstaking examination of mental states, and coordination from third-party informants." Top-down meant cursory reliance on symptom checklists. "The manual," said McHugh and Slavney, "promotes a rote-driven, essentially rule-of-thumb approach" [39]. One wouldn't actually have to be a psychiatrist, or a physician, to use it.

DSM-III-R and DSM-IV

New editions of DSM now began to churn out. In 1987, a mere 7 years after the original DSM-III, Spitzer edited a revised edition, called DSM-III-R [40]. The justification, again, was to be in lockstep with a forthcoming edition of the ICD series, ICD-10. Also, there were "new data." The changes were unremarkable, among which were converting Attention Deficit Disorder into Attention-Deficit Hyperactivity Disorder (ADHD), employing the term "mood disorders" rather than "affective disorders," and adding further confusion to the distinction, if any, between agoraphobia and panic. DSM-III-R saw the insertion of "seasonal pattern" depression into American psychiatry, following a letter to Spitzer from Thomas Wehr, chief of the Clinical Psychobiology Branch at NIMH, who mentioned that it was Norman Rosenthal's favorite diagnosis (Rosenthal was the originator, himself a sufferer) [41], and that it did seem to respond to "phototherapy" (Wehr TA to Spitzer RL, 1985 Jun 11; APA Archives, Williams papers, Research, DSM-III-R, box 4, folder "Mood"). This touched off what is, to the current writer's knowledge, the only DSM-III-R spiked epidemic: rushing to buy bright-light boxes in order to self-treat one's self-diagnosed "depression." Yet what Rosenthal called "seasonal affective disorder" was enlarged in DSM-IV to cover a whole host of affective disorders, not just "major depression." Given the almost complete lack of reliable data on seasonal affective disorder, the story is a textbook example of the influence of individual political influence upon diagnosis.

And wasn't it finally time to do something about the separation of anxiety and depression that Spitzer had engineered in 1980? In March 1985 Jack Maser, chief of the psychopathology section of NIMH, suggested to Spitzer, not that the disorders were identical, but that, "given the high incidence of depression in anxiety disorder patients, perhaps disorders [including anxiety, mania, panic, fear] should be classified as disorders of Affect." This would also make sense, he said, given that "similar pharmacologic treatment is appropriate for both depression and anxiety.... While this may be a radical departure for DSM-III-R, I believe that a case is being built for DSM-IV" (Maser JA to Spitzer RL, 1985 Mar 22; APA Archives, Williams papers, Research, DSM-III-R, box 4, "Anxiety disorders"). What actually happened is more discouraging than even the most cynical DSM-observer could have predicted: Of course mixed anxiety-depression was not included in Allen Frances's DSM-IV—it de-emphasized the primacy of anxiety—and when the drafters of DSM-5 did in fact encompass the mixed version in an early draft, they were forced to withdraw it following a sustained oppositional campaign by Frances! [42] (It may be objected that in early trials the mixed diagnosis had a low rate of agreement among diagnosticians. Yet this merely demonstrates that physicians diagnose what they are accustomed to looking for, and the mixed version had been gone from psychiatry for 30 years. One may be sure that, in 1939, if similar trials had been run for "hysteria," the inter-rater reliability would have been very high.)

In any event, DSM-III-R was merely a holding action because as early as 1979, even before the publication of DSM-III, the APA Board, their noses bloodied by Spitzer and his anti-psychoanalytic antics, had decided they wanted to move right on to DSM-IV. (Robb J to Work HH, memo, 1979 5 Oct; APA Archives, Medical Director's Office, range 37, box D-1, folder, "DSM-IV, 1979.") And they later chose as leader for DSM-IV Allen Frances, who in 1991 became the chair of psychiatry at Duke University. Frances, 52 in 1994 when DSM-IV appeared, had been trained as an analyst, and as late as 1981 was advocating the incorporation of psychoanalytic perspectives [43]. As editor of DSM-IV, however, he showed no particular allegiance to Freud's doctrines. In fact, he did not really regard his editorship of DSM as his finest moment, saying later, "In reality, I was never particularly proud of my work on DSM-IV, nor did I feel it was much of a contribution to psychiatry.... I realized well before accepting the appointment that descriptive psychiatry had reached its limits of usefulness and that the best we could hope to accomplish was to 'do no harm,' come as close to ICD-10 as possible, and establish a high standard of empirical proof so as to avoid arbitrary changes" [44]. Indeed, the last thing DSM-IV set out to do was demolish any of the DSM-III creations such as "major depression" or "schizophrenia." If anything, by reviving the diagnosis of "bipolar II," which meant depression plus hypomania, they made the diagnosis of bipolar disorder easier to get into, and the volume was partly responsible for the epidemic of "bipolar" that began to sweep psychiatry. The volume also launched the epidemic of "Asperger's disorder," supposedly mild cases of autism that began to sweep the pediatric world.

DSM-5 and Beyond

As the genesis and content of DSM-5 are considered elsewhere in this volume, it will be remarked here only that hopes were high as DSM-5 approached. One clinician wrote to a psychopharmacology listserv in 2008, "When I am sitting in clinic at 4 pm on a Tuesday afternoon, trying to make decisions on whether to medicate, what to prescribe, and what else to do, I would like a DSM that makes sense of what I am actually seeing in the clinic. When I look at drug studies, I don't see my patients. When I see DSM-V, I would like to see my patients" (Communication to a psychopharmacology listserv 2008 Feb 28[1]). Spirits are divided on the extent to which DSM-5 has realized this objective.

---

[1] Author not identified in accordance with the ground rules of the listserv.

Some problems have not been sorted out. One is whether specific psychiatric diseases really exist or whether everything is pretty well a much of a muchness, separated mainly by degrees of severity. Robert Kendell at Edinburgh and Assen Jablensky at the University of Western Australia were critical of the disease model. They argued in 2003 that the model "implicitly assumed that psychiatric disorders are discrete entities and that the role of validity criteria is to determine whether a putative disorder, such as 'good-prognosis schizophrenia' or paranoia, is a valid entity in its own right or a mild form or variant of some other entity." Maybe all the "disorders might merge into one another with no natural boundary in between," known as "points" or "zones" of rarity [45]. Moreover, they say that, "At present there is little evidence that most contemporary psychiatric diagnoses are valid, because they are still defined by syndromes that have not been demonstrated to have natural boundaries" [45]. This is a weighty objection to DSM-style thinking, particularly since the disorder-as-disease method has not acquired a particularly good track record: Paula Clayton and coworkers discovered in 1992 that, on 7-year followup, only 237 of 500 patients retained the same DSM diagnosis [46].

There is a response to this, yet it is one that does not come readily to the lips of the DSM disease-designers, because the entities that do seem to possess legitimate disease status have made it into DSM only with reluctance on the drafters' part. Melancholia and catatonia both meet the criteria for disease status, melancholia because biological markers exist for it [47]—the nec plus ultra of nosology—and catatonia because it responds to treatment in a highly differential manner (to convulsive therapy and to benzodiazepines), in a way that the diseases with which it might be confused, namely schizophrenia and encephalitis, do not [48]. At present, there is a good deal of interest in what one might think of as "the three ugly stepsisters": melancholia, catatonia, and hebephrenia. These are major disorders that have only a toehold, if that, in DSM: Melancholia was dismissed out of hand in DSM-5 as a separate entity, while catatonia was largely accepted though not as a disease of its own. Thus the question is not whether diseases or spectrums are the ideal classifying principles, but which conditions are real diseases and which require further thought.

What does the future of the DSM series hold in store, if in fact it has a future and does not collapse under the assault of collective disbelief? Will we see a return to *authoritative pronouncements* by colossal senior figures, such as Kraepelin, whose wisdom and experience it is impossible to gainsay? One might also ask, Have we reached the limits of *consensus nosology*, with its potpourri of artifactual diagnoses that do not seem to correspond to natural phenotypes? It may be that proper application of the *medical model*, with its accompanying processes of careful delimitation of symptoms, verification, and validation, offers hope yet. Maybe the medical model will help us in DSM-6 destroy the firewall between mood disorders and psychosis, a firewall that has separated "major depression" from "schizophrenia," comparable within the humoral medicine of yore to keeping black bile separate from yellow bile. In the research community, voices are already being heard in favor of demolishing the "dichotomous" classification that Emil Kraepelin originated and that DSM continues to perpetuate [49].

The consensus method involved horse-trading diagnoses to reach agreement: "We'll take away Don Klein's hysteroid dysphoria but piece him off with panic as a disease separate from anxiety." This is the kind of transaction that was customary among the DSM-III disease designers [32]. Yet such negotiation was heavily focused upon phenomenology, the signs and symptoms of the present illness, and gave little role to biochemical markers, family history, or the patient's personal history. It lacked what Bernard Carroll has called "syndromal depth... the texture one gets when salient information like your patient's past episodes and family history are considered in addition to the list of allowable symptoms" [50]. In melancholic depression, for example, psychiatrists over the last 100 years have believed in a characteristic despairing slump. (Aubrey Lewis said, "The posture is drooping and slack for the most part" [51].) This is difficult to specify in a list of operational criteria but is nonetheless real and the experienced clinician will at once recognize it [52]. How does one horse-trade this kind of information in a committee? Either it is science or it isn't.

Yet such scientific ratiocination is premature. The DSM series is more a cultural than a scientific document. In 2000 Spitzer agreed to an interviewer's assertion that DSM had become "a cultural event." Spitzer said, "It's amazing. I guess it defines things. Why do people get so upset when they have arguments about diagnosis? I guess because it defines what is the reality" [53].

Acknowledgments For comments on an earlier version, I am grateful to Bernard Carroll and Max Fink.

References

1. American College of Neuropsychopharmacology. In the beginning.... The origin of the American College of Neuropsychopharmacology. Brentwood, TN: ACNP; 1990.
2. Pinel P. Traité médico-philosophique sur l'aliénation mentale. 2nd ed. Paris: Brosson; 1809.
3. Heinroth FCA. Lehrbuch der Störungen des Seelenlebens. Leipzig: Vogel; 1818.
4. Bell LV. On a form of disease resembling some advanced stages of mania and fever, but so contradistinguished from any ordinarily observed or described combination of symptoms, as to render it probable that it may be an overlooked and hitherto unrecorded malady. Am J Insanity. 1849;6(2):97–127, 99.
5. Delasiauve L. Du diagnostic différentiel de la lypémanie. Ann Méd Psychol. 1851;(3):380–442, 380.
6. Kraepelin E. Compendium der Psychiatrie. Leipzig: Abel; 1883.
7. Kraepelin E. Psychiatrie: ein kurzes Lehrbuch für Studierende und Ärzte. 8th ed. Leipzig: Barth; 1909–1915.
8. Gaupp R. Die Frage der kombinierten Psychosen. Zeits Neurol Psychiatry. 1926;76(1):73–80, 77–8.
9. Bleuler E, Jung CG. Komplexe und Krankheitsursachen bei Dementia praecox. Zentralbl Nervenheilk Psychiatr. 1908;19:220–7.
10. Kraepelin E. Psychiatrie: ein kurzes Lehrbuch für Studierende und Ärzte. 6th ed. Leipzig: Barth; 1899.
11. Kraepelin E. Die Abgrenzung der Paranoia. Allg Zeits Psychiatr. 1894;50:1080–1.
12. Lewis A. "Endogenous" and "exogenous": a useful dichotomy? Psychol Med. 1971;1(3):191–6.

13. Stengel E. Classification of mental disorders. Bull World Health Organ. 1959;21(4–5):601–63.
14. Menninger WC. Psychiatric nomenclature. J Nerv Ment Dis. 1946;104(2):180–99.
15. Fink M. Interview. In: Ban TA, editor. An oral history of neuropsychopharmacology: the first fifty years; peer interviews, vol. 9. Brentwood, TN: ACNP; 2011. p. 76.
16. World Health Organization. Manual of the international statistical classification of diseases, injuries and causes of death. 6th revision [later known as ICD-6] 2 volumes. Geneva: WHO; 1948–49.
17. American Psychiatric Association. Diagnostic and statistical manual of mental disorders. Washington, DC: APA; 1952.
18. Klein DF, Fink M. Psychiatric reaction patterns to imipramine. Am J Psychiatry. 1962; 119(5):432–8.
19. Müller C. Lexikon der Psychiatrie. Berlin: Springer; 1973. p. 409–15.
20. Lambert P. Discussion. In: Bradley PB, Deniker P, Raduoco-Thomas C, editors. Neuro-psychopharmacology: proceedings of the first international congress of neuro-psychopharmacology, Rome, September 1958. Amsterdam: Elsevier; 1959. p. 212.
21. American Psychiatric Association. DSM-II: diagnostic and statistical manual of mental disorders. 2nd ed. Washington, DC: APA; 1968.
22. Kendell RE, Cooper JE, Gourlay AJ, Copeland JRM, Sharpe L, Gurland BJ. Diagnostic criteria of American and British psychiatrists. Arch Gen Psychiatry. 1971;25(2):123–30.
23. Frank J. Discussion comment. In: Zubin J, Freyhan F, editors. Disorders of mood. Baltimore: Johns Hopkins Press; 1972. p. 30.
24. Katz M, Williams TA, Shield JA. Recent advances in the psychobiology of the depressive illnesses. Proceedings of a workshop hosted by the College of William and Mary in Virginia, April 30 through May 2, 1969. National Institute of Mental Health, Division of Extramural Research Programs, Clinical Research branch. Washington, DC: Superintendent of Documents, US Government Printing Office; 1972.
25. Weissman M. Interview. Gerald Klerman and psychopharmacology. In: Healy D, editor. The psychopharmacologists, vol. 2. London: Altman; 1998. p. 521–42, 530.
26. Clayton PJ. Interview. In: Ban TA, editor. An oral history of neuropsychopharmacology: the first fifty years; peer interviews, vol. 7. Brentwood, TN: ACNP; 2011. p. 99.
27. Henn FA. Interview. In: Ban TA, editor. An oral history of neuropsychopharmacology: the first fifty years; peer interviews, vol. 8. Brentwood, TN: ACNP; 2011. p. 154.
28. Feighner JP, Robins E, Guze SB, Woodruff RA, Winokur G, Muñoz R. Diagnostic criteria for use in psychiatric research. Arch Gen Psychiatry. 1972;26(1):57–63.
29. Katz MM. Interview. In: Ban TA, editor. An oral history of neuropsychopharmacology: the first fifty years; peer interviews, vol. 9. Brentwood, TN: ACNP; 2011. p. 200.
30. Shorter E. Bipolar disorder in historical perspective. In: Parker G, editor. Bipolar II disorder: modeling, measuring and managing. 2nd ed. Cambridge, UK: Cambridge University Press; 2012. p. 1–9.
31. Spitzer RL, Endicott J, Robins E, Kuriansky J, Gurland B. Preliminary report of the reliability of research diagnostic criteria applied to psychiatric case records. In: Sudilovsky A, Gershon S, Beer B, editors. Predictability in psychopharmacology: preclinical and clinical correlations. New York: Raven; 1975. p. 1–47.
32. Shorter E. How everyone became depressed: the rise and fall of the nervous breakdown. New York: Oxford University Press; 2013.
33. Spitzer RL, Endicott J, Robins E. Research diagnostic criteria. Arch Gen Psychiatry. 1978;35(6):773–82.
34. Klein DF. Interview. In: Ban TA, editor. An oral history of neuropsychopharmacology: the first fifty years; peer interviews, vol. 9. Brentwood, TN: ACNP; 2011. p. 214.
35. Klerman GL, Endicott J, Spitzer R, Hirschfeld RMA. Neurotic depressions: a systematic analysis of multiple criteria and meanings. Am J Psychiatry. 1979;136(1):57–61.
36. Rudorfer MV, Clayton PJ. Depression, dementia and dexamethasone suppression [letter]. Am J Psychiatry. 1981;138(5):701.
37. Healy D, editor. The psychopharmacologists, vol. 2. London: Altman; 1998. p. 555.

38. Taylor MA, Vaidya NA. Descriptive psychopathology: the signs and symptoms of behavioral disorders. Cambridge, UK: Cambridge University Press; 2009.
39. McHugh PR, Slavney PR. Mental illness—comprehensive evaluation or checklist? N Engl J Med. 2012;366(20):1853–5, 1854.
40. American Psychiatric Association. Diagnostic and statistical manual of mental disorders (third edition—revised): DSM-III-R. Washington, DC: APA; 1987.
41. Rosenthal NE, Sack DA, Gillin JC, Lewy AJ, Goodwin FK, Davenport Y, et al. Seasonal affective disorder: a description of the syndrome and preliminary findings with light therapy. Arch Gen Psychiatry. 1984;41(1):72–80.
42. Frances A. Opening Pandora's box: the 19 worst suggestions for DSM-5. Psychiatric Times, 11 Feb 2010.
43. Frances A, Cooper AM. Descriptive and dynamic psychiatry: a perspective on DSM-III. Am J Psychiatry. 1981;138(9):1198–202.
44. Frances A. Dr Frances responds to Dr Carpenter: a sharp difference of opinion. Psychiatric Times, 9 Jul 2009.
45. Kendell R, Jablensky A. Distinguishing between the validity and utility of psychiatric diagnoses. Am J Psychiatry. 2003;160(1):4–12, 5, 11.
46. Clayton PJ, Guze SB, Cloninger CR, Martin RL. Unipolar depression: diagnostic inconsistency and its implications. J Affect Disord. 1992;26(2):111–6.
47. Taylor MA, Fink M. Melancholia: the diagnosis, pathophysiology, and treatment of depressive illness. Cambridge, UK: Cambridge University Press; 2006.
48. Fink M, Taylor MA. Catatonia: a clinician's guide to diagnosis and treatment. Cambridge, UK: Cambridge University Press; 2003.
49. Craddock N, Owen MJ. Rethinking psychosis: the disadvantages of a dichotomous classification now outweigh the advantages. World Psychiatry. 2007;6(2):84–91.
50. Carroll B. Comment on: as precisely as possible. In: 1 Boring old man [Internet]. http://1boringoldman.com/index.php/2011/12/05/as-precisely-as-possible/. Accessed 5 Dec 2011.
51. Parker G, Hadzi-Pavlovic D, Wilhelm K, Hickie I, Brodaty H, Boyce P, et al. Defining melancholia: properties of a refined sign-based measure. Br J Psychiatry. 1994;164(3):316–26.
52. Lewis AJ. Melancholia: a clinical survey of depressive states. J Ment Sci. 1934;80(329): 277–378, 280.
53. Spitzer R. Interview. In: Healy D, editor. The psychopharmacologists, vol. 3. London: Altman; 1998. p. 427.

Chapter 2
Considering the Economy of DSM Alternatives

John Z. Sadler

The development and release of DSM-III in 1980 [1] not only ushered in an era of descriptive diagnostic classification, but also ushered in scholarly, critical analyses of diagnostic classification systems and diagnostic practice. The reasons for these states of affairs should not be surprising. In retrospect the DSMs have served as an unique source of mental health policy: encoding the nomenclature and psychopathological constructs for all to consider, whether administrators, payers, educators, researchers, the public, or practicing clinicians [2–4]. DSM concepts have found their way into popular culture, only one of the myriad examples being the discussions of DSM concepts in patient/consumer websites, online blogs, and web-forums [5]. The dominance of the DSM as policy reference point and cultural icon has led some commentators to accuse the manuals of being hegemonic for psychiatry and mental health [6].

Remarkably, despite the intense scholarly interest in the DSMs as scientific classifications of psychopathology as well as sociocultural phenomena, little has been written about why the post-DSM-III DSMs have come to dominate American mental health. This chapter provides one historical-explanatory perspective.

The structure of the chapter is straightforward, organized into four sections. After a brief discussion of historical background and context, the second section develops the case for a sociocultural phenomenon called the "mental health medical-industrial complex" (MHMIC). The third section describes my core thesis that the MHMIC is largely responsible for the hegemony of the DSMs, to the degree that the DSMs are indeed hegemonic. The concluding section discusses the ramifications, offers some alternatives, and summarizes conclusions.

For this chapter, my intention is only to address the particular concatenation of economic conditions in the United States. To address other countries, such as

J.Z. Sadler, MD (✉)
Department of Psychiatry, The University of Texas
Southwestern Medical Center, Dallas, TX, USA
e-mail: John.Sadler@utsouthwestern.edu

J. Paris and J. Phillips (eds.), *Making the DSM-5: Concepts and Controversies*,
DOI 10.1007/978-1-4614-6504-1_2, © Springer Science+Business Media New York 2013

Europe or even the US near-neighbor, Canada, would require more work than I am capable for a single chapter. Hopefully, our international colleagues will weigh in on the question of a MHMIC in Western industrialized societies.

Historical Context

DSM-III was hugely successful after its release in 1980 [7], having been translated into over a dozen languages, becoming not just hugely influential in US clinical research and clinical practice but also a credible rival to the World Health Organization's (WHO) International Classification of Diseases (ICD), Mental and Behavioural Disorders [8] text. However, the controversies about the DSMs appeared almost immediately, with book-length discussions [3, 4, 9–16] and countless articles appearing through each iteration of the manual since, right up into the present day with DSM-5 and this current volume.

The importance and influence of the DSM have been established elsewhere (see prior references) and will be assumed for this discussion. The nosological dominance of the DSMs, however, has not gone without candidate challengers. The DSM's most serious rival is the series of classifications of mental and behavioral disorders offer by the WHO under the ICD label. Since DSM-III, however, the diagnostic administrative coding for the DSM categories and the ICD coding have agreed, under treaty arrangement, to be compatible and "cross-talk" with each other [7]. The "clinical modification" version of ICD diagnoses dictate numeric codes used in the DSM and in this context remain crucial to administrative and billing uses. The DSM authors have made practical judgments about the right fit between ICD categories and DSM categories, because the two classifications are not identical [17]. In addition to the limited comparability between the two systems, another major difference in the two manuals is the use of elaborate diagnostic criteria in the DSMs. The other substantive difference with the ICD is that it provides not just a system for coding mental and behavioral disorders, but a system of coding for *all* diseases, injuries, and handicaps, extending far beyond the circumscribed domain of mental disorders in the DSMs [8, 18, 19]. In these senses the ICD-CM Manuals are more partners than rivals to the DSMs.

Partly in reaction to dissatisfactions with DSM-II and the early discussions of DSM-III, a Task Force on Descriptive Behavioral Classification, chaired by Dr. Wilbur E. Morley, was formed by the American Psychological Association in 1977 [20] (see also [21, 22]; thanks to Roger Blashfield PhD for the original reference document). The agenda of this psychologist's Task Force, however, never got off the ground, likely due to the diverse membership of the American Psychological Association (not all of whom were even clinicians) and the enormous difficulties in building any consensus among such a large and diverse organization.

A number of investigator-initiated diagnostic systems have been developed before and after the debut of DSM-III in 1980. However, these have had circumscribed, not comprehensive, sets of categories, and while likely influential in the refinement of DSM categories and criteria, have not posed much of a threat to the overall DSM enterprise [23–25]. More recently, psychiatric geneticists and neurobiologists have explored the notion of "endophenotypes" as intermediate taxa, hopefully linking concepts between neurobiological/genetic processes and the clinical phenomenology of psychopathology [26, 27]. These, however, have not found their way as yet into an independent classification of psychopathology, and their status as criterion items for DSM-5 categories is unknown at this writing.

These latter concepts are a natural transition to the recent debut of the Research Domain Criteria (RDoC) classification promulgated by the leadership of the National Institute of Mental Health (NIMH). Arising out of psychiatric neuroscientists' dissatisfactions with the DSMs [28–30] and assimilated into the NIMH's 2008 Strategic Plan [31], the RDoC described a matrix of seven units of analysis (genes, molecules, cells, circuits, physiology, behavior, self-reports) against five domains/constructs (negative valence [emotional] systems, positive valence systems, cognitive systems, social processes, and arousal/regulatory processes) [32]. The significance of this framework for research, as well as clinical practice, has yet to be demonstrated. However, given that it is promulgated by the same institution (NIMH) that provides the greatest amount of grant support for psychiatric research in the world, one might imagine that the RDoC framework will be vigorously supported by NIMH grant-seekers (The robust conflict-of-interest issues raised by this arrangement [33] will be only acknowledged at this point, see more below).

The Military Industrial Complex

In the aftermath of a devastating World War II, and in the shadow of an expansionist Soviet totalitarian empire, US President Dwight D. Eisenhower in 1961 coined what was to be an influential trope, still familiar today. In his farewell speech from the White House, Eisenhower presented his concerns about a "military industrial complex" (see National Public Radio online, http://www.npr.org/2011/01/17/132942244/ikes-warning-of-military-expansion-50-years-later). This quote from that speech sums up the concept:

> This conjunction of an immense military establishment and a large arms industry is new in the American experience. The **total influence—economic, political, even spiritual**—is felt in every city, every State house, every office of the Federal government. We recognize the imperative need for this development. Yet we **must not fail to comprehend its grave implications**. Our toil, resources and livelihood are all involved; so is the very structure of our society.
>
> In the councils of government, **we must guard against the acquisition of unwarranted influence, whether sought or unsought, by the military industrial complex.** The potential for the disastrous rise of misplaced power exists and will persist.
>
> We must never let the weight of this combination endanger our liberties or democratic processes. We should take nothing for granted. Only an **alert and knowledgeable citizenry** can complete the proper meshing of the huge industrial and military machinery of defense with our peaceful methods and goals, so that security and liberty may prosper together [34] (p. 1035; boldface emphasis added).

The basic idea is that the United States' huge investment and dependence upon a colossal military industry can exert undue influence on the political process. However, such dependence can also transform our thinking, as Eisenhower suggests through his inclusion of "spiritual" influence to his list of concerns. Importantly, he notes that the undue influence of the complex can be intentional or unintended, and only an "alert and knowledgeable citizenry" can provide a check against these influences.

Almost five decades later, a former Chief of the NIMH (1991–1993), Bernadine Healy MD, opined in the *US News & World Report*:

> If only we had remembered Eisenhower's less famous second warning: that **"public policy could itself become the captive of a scientific-technological elite"** in which the **"power of money is ever present."** He feared elites would dominate the nation's scholars **by virtue of their federal employment** or **their control over large research grants**. Eisenhower was thinking about the solitary tinkerer overrun by task forces of scientists, but his instincts were prescient [35] (no pages, boldface emphasis added).

Dr. Healy was concerned that a "medical-industrial complex" had arisen. Like the Military Industrial Complex, she claimed our health and scientific policy was unduly influenced by these moneyed "elites" who could frame the very terms of scientific discourse and marginalize all alternative thinkers, whether "solitary tinkerers" or small collectives (see also [36]).

Admittedly, these kinds of interpretations of social processes are difficult to establish with a scientific standard of evidence. Nevertheless, the remainder of this paper will argue that Healy's concern was timely and perhaps even more apparent in the fields of psychiatry and mental health. I will provide a descriptive analysis of our current social state of affairs in the United States to defend this idea. I intend that the self-evident nature of Eisenhower's and Healy's vision will manifest through this descriptive analysis.

The Mental Health-Medical-Industrial Complex

The MHMIC is an analogue to the medical-industrial complex described by Healy. However, as the mental health system encompasses its own distinctive domains, only partially overlapping with the medical corpus, I sketch the components of a MHMIC below. Through comprehending the whole through its components and their interactions with each other, one can see the relatively exclusive and exclusionary hold the MHMIC has on not just diagnostic considerations, but the mental health field as a whole.

Regarding the dominance of the DSM, my thesis is simple: The DSM has prevailed because it has, on balance, served its function in the MHMIC, whose monolithic influences on funding, public policy, and the social discourse on mental illness reinforces the DSM's stability and success. This thesis has several corollaries:

> Corollary (1): Economic reductionism. Most pertinently to DSM-5, to the degree that DSM-5 conforms to the functional needs (e.g., continued economic dominance) of the

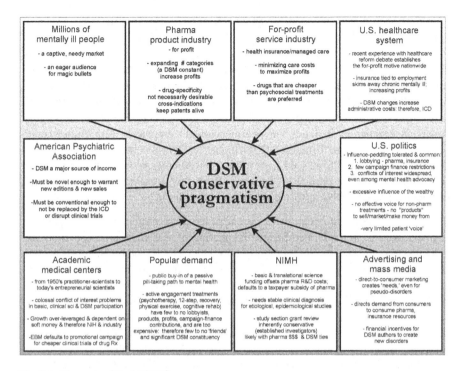

Fig. 2.1 Elements of the MHMIC

MHMIC, the DSMs will continue to flourish and dominate. However, as will be discussed in the concluding section, this is not a foregone conclusion at this moment in DSM-5 development (summer 2012) and before its completion and estimated release in 2013.

Corollary (2): Shaping the scientific frame. Alternatives which do not fit into the MHMIC will be squeezed out (marginalized) by MHMIC-friendly scientific funding, peer review, and publication forces.

Corollary (3): Medicalization. "Medicalization describes a process by which human problems come to be defined and treated as medical problems" [37]. With this understanding, the MHMIC promulgates a de facto mode of thinking where all mental distress, disordered or otherwise, is a technological problem which can be addressed by the development of commercial products and sold to professionals and the public as therapies or solutions (see [38]).

Figure 2.1 sketches ten component-elements of the MHMIC, and I will discuss each of the components, their identity and interactions with other components, as my next step. The frame for this discussion could be called "DSM conservative pragmatism." Under this rubric, "conservative" means resistant to change in the general sense, not in the political-ideological sense of partisanship [39]. "Pragmatism" means that pragmatic (along with scientific) considerations are the primary reference point for changes to the DSMs. The figure suggests that the elements of the MHMIC "conspire" to stabilize a DSM with minimal changes.

Element 1: Millions of mentally ill people. The business appeal of tens of millions of people needing a product is transparent. However, having tens of millions of people who are in varying needs of extreme need or *desperation* for those products multiplies said business opportunities and offers an extraordinary market. However, the exceptionalism of the mental healthcare market is further multiplied by the provision of funding through insurance and public assistance so that even people who could not otherwise afford mental health products can obtain them. It should be no surprise that the pharmaceutical and medical device industries are among the biggest businesses in the United States. The 2011 Forbes 500 listing of the largest American companies includes ten pharmaceutical companies (http://money.cnn.com/magazines/fortune/fortune500/2011/industries/21/index.html). Five of those (Johnson & Johnson, Pfizer, Eli Lilly, Amgen, and Abbott) are in the *Fortune* magazine 2011 top 50 most profitable companies list (http://money.cnn.com/magazines/fortune/fortune500/2011/performers/companies/profits/).

Element 2: Pharmaceutical industry. As one of the most influential and competitive business markets in the United States, the pharmaceutical companies (pharma) are obligated to maximize profits for their shareholders. Not bound by any professional ethics, but only by governmental constraints of a regulated free market and by company duty to stockholders, one component aim of pharma is to expand markets. In that regard, an ongoing commitment from American psychiatry to increase the number of categories of mental disorders is a valuable, perhaps essential, contribution to this expansionist agenda. So far, each revision of the DSM has added new categories and/or subcategories of disorders [4, 7]. Moreover, pharma likely benefits from the "atheoretical" descriptive approach to diagnosis, in that atheoreticism contributes to the potential for cross-indications (cross-indications are use of the same compound for different diagnostic categories, such as using SSRIs for both depression and anxiety disorders). Off-label use (physician prescription of compounds without FDA approval for particular disorders) also contributes to expanding markets for products.

In contrast, the development of theoretically rich, highly specific treatments for singular conditions limit marketability and profits through reducing the potential for cross-indications and perhaps off-label use, in addition to limiting the numbers of treatment-eligible patients. Finally, the DSMs' trend toward categorizing conditions which overlap with ordinary life experience, like shyness [40] or grief [41] maintains an economic expansionist model from which the pharmaceutical industry (not to overlook psychiatrists) may profit. In these senses the pharmaceutical industry and the DSMs are de facto "partners" [42–44].

Element 3: For-profit service industry. In this setting, I mean the "for-profit service industry" to refer to health insurance and related funding sources of health care, as well as managed care organizations which regulate spending for health care. Because in the United States this industry, which is another huge conglomerate of businesses, is also mostly oriented to maximizing profits, cost controls on the clinical-service delivery side are a preeminent concern. A primary mechanism for maximizing profits is minimizing care costs, as under the insurance model, customers pay-in to a pool of funds from which both services are paid for and profits for the company are generated. Simply put, the less the service industry pays for care, the more money they make.

This incentive to minimize care reaches equilibrium when cost- and care-cutting cross thresholds of clinical adequacy and tolerability with physicians and patients, generating protest, and threatening a loss of market share through moving care contracts elsewhere. Because of the service industry's interests in maximizing value per dollar spent, drug therapy becomes a cheap alternative to psychosocial therapies which are service-intensive and therefore more expensive [45]. DSM categories offer conditions which fit easily into the clinical-trial format, compared to psychosocial treatments, for which meaningful placebo/control groups are difficult and expensive to develop. Hence clinical-trial-friendly DSM categories enter into a mutually reinforcing arrangement where industry supports clinical trials, the service industry gets cheap treatments, and DSM developers can benefit from industry clinical-trial contracts, consulting arrangements, and the like [42–44].

Element 4: US healthcare system. As the recent debate over President Obama's Affordable Care Act has echoed past US failures to provide comprehensive health care for all, the idea of a nonprofit, single-payer US healthcare system has not been politically feasible [46–49]. The reasons for this state of affairs are complex. Alexis de Tocqueville described American individualism (as opposed to European collectivism) in the middle of the nineteenth century in his *Democracy in America* [50]. Scholars have debated the US national character ever since [51]. Blendon and Benson [46] note that over the past 50 years, Americans have generally been satisfied with their personal healthcare arrangements, they are distrustful of the federal government involvement in health care, and consistently oppose single-payer plans. However, the economic and political power of the service industry and pharma alone present an extraordinary lobbying force on US policy [52, 53], compounded recently by changes in campaign-finance regulation (see next section and section on "Advertising and Mass Media"). The degree to which these lobbying and advertising campaigns contributed to public viewpoints is difficult to determine. In any case, US healthcare will likely remain a for-profit business enterprise for the foreseeable future. The role of the DSMs in the US healthcare system per se is largely administrative, and diluted in effect because of the common use of ICD-Clinical Modification coding. However, to the degree that DSM changes are made, this may increase administrative costs, and therefore constitute a demand for relative "conservatism" when DSM revisions are made.

Element 5: US politics. The above vectors interact with aspects of US politics, aspects which in recent years have compounded the power and influence of the MHMIC. US politics maintains the political power of corporate wealth, through the mechanisms of lobbying (see section "Advertising and Mass Media") and, most recently, campaign financing by the wealthy. The recent upholding of unlimited private funding for election campaigns in the US Supreme Court [54] further strengthens the potential for influence-peddling by the kind of "moneyed elites" that worried Eisenhower and Healy. Writing for the dissenting US Supreme Court *Citizens United* opinion, Justice Stevens summarized: "A democracy cannot function effectively when its constituent members believe laws are being bought and sold" [54]. In concluding, Justice Stevens notes:

At bottom, the Court's opinion is thus a rejection of the common sense of the American people, who have recognized a need to prevent corporations from undermining self-government since the founding, and who have fought against the distinctive corrupting potential of corporate electioneering since the days of Theodore Roosevelt. It is a strange time to repudiate that common sense. While American democracy is imperfect, few outside the majority of this Court would have thought its flaws included a dearth of corporate money in politics [54].

In comparison to the corporate wealth of the healthcare service industries and pharma, the political powers of the mentally ill, their families, and even American psychiatry are feeble at best. Their ability to advocate for themselves is limited, and today in the United States such advocacy is primarily done by "mental health advocacy groups."

The corrupting potential of corporate money is present even within mental health advocacy groups. In 2009 the *New York Times* noted that the National Alliance for the Mentally Ill's support from pharma was nearly 75% over the past 3 years [55]. NAMI still accepts large pharma donations, as can be seen on its website [56]. For first quarter 2012, 58% of NAMI's support came from pharma [56]. Mental Health America's 2010 Annual Report does not list dollar amounts of corporate gifts, but does list pharmaceutical companies by their financial range of donations. For the highest level, $100,000 and above, Astra-Zeneca, Bristol-Myers Squibb, Eli Lilly, and Sunovion account for all contributors but one; for their second largest category, $50,000–99,999, Forest, Merck, and Novartis are three of five contributors [57].

The openness of US politics to influence-peddling diminishes political opportunity for resources for non-pharmacological treatment interventions. Psychosocial treatments like the psychotherapies, recovery-oriented peer interventions, and the like have no commercial product to sell, no corporate donations to politicians, and no lobbyists advocating for them on Capitol Hill. Subsequently, their "voice" in setting treatment, reimbursement, and research priorities is trivial in comparison to the pharmaceutical and medical device industry.

Element 6: Advertising and mass media. The use of advertising and mass media in promoting medical products has reached unprecedented levels over nearly 30 years since the FDA permitted direct-to-consumer marketing of medications and other medical products in the early 1980s [58]. Such advertising, like all medical advertising, is intended to create or divert demand for products that may, or may not be, necessary for health or well-being. In the mental health arena, where the demarcation between normal and pathological experience/behavior is often not sharp, such marketing can create public demand for pseudo-disorders, as discussed in depth by such recent scholarly publications as *The Loss of Sadness: How Psychiatry Transformed Normal Sorrow into Depressive Disorder* by Allan V. Horwitz and Jerome C. Wakefield [41] and Christopher Lane's *Shyness: How Normal Behavior Became a Sickness* [40].

In his eye-opening exposé of the use of public relations in promoting industry interests (*Deadly Spin*), Wendell Potter [59], a former head of communications for health insurance giant CIGNA, details the systematic and extensive mobilization of the medical service industry to lobby for the political defeat of the Affordable Care

Act. Potter paints a picture of a corporate lobby spending millions to defeat "Obamacare" using advertising, obfuscation, and misinformation as its tools. Today Potter runs a website (http://wendellpotter.com/) that is a hub for reporting of all kinds of medical influence-peddling. While the actual impact of such clandestine public-relations campaigns is difficult to ascertain, the ubiquity of US political advertising suggests substantial impact.

The massive promotional efforts to the public by industry likely both create public attitudes toward mental health treatment as well as reinforce industry-favorable prejudices, factors that will be discussed in Element 8 below.

Element 7: NIMH. From its beginnings in 1949, the NIMH was authorized and funded by Congress to develop an extramural research grant and intramural research program into the causes of, diagnosis of, and treatments for mental illnesses [60]. In the early years of NIMH, under the leadership of Robert Felix, NIMH also stimulated the development of alternatives to the state hospitals, mostly through the development of community clinics and preventative programs which developed in virtually every state by the mid-1950s. The NIMH also offered training grants to develop competent new clinicians. However, in the ensuing decades the commitment to community, prevention, and training faded, and the contemporary model for the NIMH came to replace it, speeded by the discovery of new psychopharmacological treatments in the 1950s and 1960s [61, 62]. By the 1990s "Decade of the Brain," the NIMH came to focus primarily upon funding basic neuroscience, genetic, and related research aimed at finding molecules and biomechanisms suitable for development of drug or other biomedical treatments. The NIMH mission of funding clinical trials to establish efficacy—the mission that was largely responsible for the Food & Drug Administration (FDA) approval of lithium therapy for manic-depressive illness—came to be shunted to the pharmaceutical companies, who increasingly funded clinical trials for their own products, both serving the need to establish efficacy for FDA approval purposes, but also to supply marketing rhetoric in the guise of scientific data. The sham nature of many pharma-sponsored clinical trials was exposed in the early 2000s, when the widespread suppression of negative clinical trials was discovered and made public [63–65]. These trends contributed to increased scrutiny of industry-sponsored clinical trials through a mandatory online registry, http://www.clinicaltrials.gov/.

Today, NIMH funding is built around individual Institutes and Centers, whose funding is a complex combination of the Director's whim, Congressional agendas, and the demand of investigators [33]. The de facto arrangement of taxpayer-supported basic science through NIMH with clinical trials referred to the pharmaceutical industry for sponsorship amounts to a taxpayer subsidy of the pharmaceutical industry's research and development. The NIMH does the basic and translational science, whose results in the public sphere can be appropriated by the pharmaceutical companies in the development of new therapeutic agents. In the meantime, fundamental and important questions regarding health services, psychosocial treatments, conceptual issues, public health, and patient initiatives remain marginally funded [33].

Regarding the NIMH and the DSMs, two additional comments should be made. First, the system of grant review by peer scientists ("study sections") is an inherently conservative process. That is, only established and successful (by NIMH funding standards) investigators are invited to serve on grant review committees. Such investigators, having based their careers on DSM categories and criteria, are unlikely to look favorably at truly innovative mechanisms of diagnosis, so entrenched are the DSMs in the clinical research infrastructure over the past 30 years. Indeed, the promulgation of the RDoC concept by the NIMH itself raises questions about an intent to break the hold the DSMs have on clinical/translational extramural research submissions. In a related vein, as Cosgrove and colleagues have suggested through their identification of widespread conflicts of interest among DSM and APA clinical treatment guidelines thought leaders [42–44], pharmaceutical funding of said thought leaders may well further entrench DSM categories as any alternative poses an unproven and unforeseeable risk to pharma interests. The second point is more straightforward: clinical and epidemiological studies, in order to maintain more generalizable findings, need standard and stable sets of diagnostic categories and criteria [66, 67] which also likely contribute to the stability of DSM use among NIMH study sections.

Element 8: Popular demand. Research into "health literacy" (understanding of medicine's capabilities, limitations, and the role of self-care and prevention) has indicated that for the public, health literacy is low [68–73]. The promulgation of advertisements and promotions of pill-taking as the solution to all ills has resulted in the public buy-in of a passive model of mental health—one need only take a pill to get better [74]. In contrast, mental health treatments that could be characterized as "active" or "engaged" include psychotherapies, 12-step programs, physical exercise, cognitive rehabilitation, to name a few. The irony here is, despite the strong evidence-bases for efficacy for many of them, these active/engaged treatment modalities generally have no lobby, no corporate investment, no potential for profit-generation, no campaign-finance contributions, or other mechanisms to breach the fence of the MHMIC. Moreover, they are generally more expensive than passive, product-based therapies, and therefore have few to no "friends" among the DSM constituencies with their pharma industry support. Descriptive categories suitable to these modalities of treatment may not exist in the DSM approach. These modalities may be tied to their own theoretical formulation and relevant nomenclature.

Element 9: Academic medical centers (AMCs). Reading the history of psychopharmacology provided by David Healy [61, 62] provides a useful window into the history of the physician-investigator in AMCs. In the 1950s and 1960s physician investigators often performed their research in the context of everyday clinical work in clinics and hospitals. We might call this model of clinical research that of the "physician-scientist." That is, these clinicians performed their research with their own patients, doing studies that today would be called "descriptive studies" or occasional trials of compounds with limited controls. Because the research ethics review (IRB) infrastructure that regulates human subjects research today didn't exist until the late 1980s, physician-scientists had few constraints in performing their work other than their own consciences. However, over the remaining decades of the twentieth century, clinical research came to be increasingly a part of AMCs: conglomerates of medical schools, teaching hospitals, and other clinical schools and services. Over decades, a shift in the character of the physician-scientist changed as AMCs changed, both becoming more dependent upon "soft money"—salary support from grants and contracts with distinct startup and completion cycles. This shift became compounded as AMCs expanded their financial bases from state support, donations, and clinical revenues, becoming more and more dependent upon the soft money of grants and contracts [75, 76]. AMCs became highly "leveraged" institutions, unable to support their faculties with hard and reliable sources of support, and vulnerable to budget shortfalls in the case of failed grant-and contract-winning. Bringing in money has come to characterize the successful academic physician, and a more apt description for today's clinical investigator is "physician-entrepreneur." This shift from hard to soft money then provided the social background for the huge conflict-of-interest dilemmas that have faced AMCs over the past two decades (see [77] for a detailed review).

From the DSM perspective, concerns have been raised by Lisa Cosgrove and colleagues [42–44] about the financial relationships and undue influence of medical industry on DSM panelists, most of whom are AMC academics, subject to severe soft-money generation pressures. The over-leveraged status of American AMCs makes them beholden to NIH and industry for their very survival; making the potential for compromising their traditional missions (education, patient care, research) equally severe.

The MHMIC influence even extends into movements like evidence-based medicine (EBM) [78, 79], which intends to build into medical practice a more rigorous use of scientific evidence. However, if the scientific evidence is unduly influenced by financial interests, the rigor of the science is questionable and the utility of the evidence is in question. In a 2007 article considering the applicability of EBM to psychiatry, Mona Gupta [80] argues that the particular complexity of mental disorders does not fit the parameters of EBM. Given the difficulty with doing controlled trials of psychosocial treatment interventions, and with clinical trials being the principal EBM criterion of evidence quality, the prospects of psychosocial treatments competing successfully for an "evidence base" are curtailed. Instead, passive treatment modalities like medications become the default prime candidate for evidence-based treatment. Medication treatments dominate EBM reviews not because they are necessarily superior, but because medications have the MHMIC economic support behind them to generate a strong evidence base. In psychiatry, EBM defaults to evidence-based psychopharmacology, and the over-leveraged AMC systems are the platform in which evidence-based psychopharmacology is promulgated, using DSM categories as an essential instrument.

Element 10: American Psychiatric Association. It is widely acknowledged that the DSMs are a source of income to the American Psychiatric Association to the tune of tens of millions of dollars a year [4]. Psychologist Roger Blashfield, in his Taxonomy of Psychopathology blog, estimates that DSM-IV earned between $5 million and $6 million dollars a year between 2005 and 2011, based upon APA Treasurer's reports [81]. Given the size of this financial interest, the promulgation of the DSMs has to be partly motivated by profit interests [4]. The degree to which profitability determines DSM policy remains a secret of the APA leadership.

The financial power of the DSM poses tough decisions for that APA leadership. The manual must be novel enough to warrant new purchases on a regular basis, through new editions, but not be so frequently reissued that sales expectations are diminished through disinterest. However, the DSM must be conventional enough as to not lose its dominant place in market share, as well as not tarnish its relationship with the ICD. Given the substantial amounts of income generated by the manual, perhaps it is fair to say that a proper balance of stability and innovation is important to the APA's financial status. So still another economic incentive serves to maintain the DSM in its powerful position.

Ramifications and Conclusions

A friend and colleague at the APA symposium in which these ideas were introduced noted that my presentation was "depressing." To conclude that the DSM is impossibly corrupt and flawed would be easy, as would be to demonize the MHMIC as an evil to be demolished. That would make as much sense as saying investment in the military industrial complex is wholly evil; and only then if you were an ideologically committed pacifist. I should acknowledge that the MHMIC provides the only credible resource for developing, testing, and promulgating products to help doctors help patients. What concerned Eisenhower and Bernadine Healy was the idea that the "moneyed elites" have profound potential to compromise other important values and missions for the country. Similarly, the moneyed elites have profound potential to corrupt other important values and missions for psychiatry, mental health, and their affiliated institutions.

Personally, I believe that the MHMIC-related compromise of other important mental health values is ongoing and increased in recent years, making for the most severe negative compromises I have witnessed in my lifetime. For instance, the withholding of negative clinical trials by pharma in past decades has thrown much, perhaps most, synthetic wisdom about psychopharmacological efficacy into question. Knowing, with a reasonable amount of certainty, what drugs work in psychiatry is an overwhelming task suitable only to an investigative scholar with open access to government, private enterprise, the scientific literature, and huge amounts of time and money. In an earlier paper challenging the NIMH/NIH investment in psychiatric molecular genetics, I suggested that the hundreds of millions of dollars in research investment in the field are questionable given the many research questions that, if answered with funding, could make an impact on mental health care immediately. These research questions, however, have to do with psychosocial treatments, patient attitudes, conceptual issues, and access to care questions that don't have products attached and therefore have little to no political influence [33]. The MHMIC machine that seeks magic bullets to cure psychiatric illness has been given much more than its due. The magic-bullet approach to psychiatric treatment has continued to be vigorously funded with mediocre results as measured in terms of actual improvements in care, even according to the scientists that perform this research, as well as the NIMH [31, 33]. I agree that we "must guard against the acquisition of unwarranted influence" but that unwarranted influence is already in historically established play. American psychiatry is behind the curve in guarding against unwarranted influence.

Regarding the DSM, what surprised me in my analysis for this chapter was that I came in agreeing with many critics about the "hegemony" of the DSMs, and that somehow the APA and the DSM architects were invested in maintaining that hegemony. While the latter may or may not be true, I now perceive the DSMs as simply cogs in a much bigger economic machine, the MHMIC, whose drivers and self-interested incentives lock-in many of the features that make the DSM "hegemonic."

What to do is easy to list in the abstract, and could be addressed for each of my ten elements of influence. What can be easily listed, however, is tremendously difficult to execute. For Element 1, millions of mentally ill people, education efforts to address the contributions and limitations of somatic treatments could be helpful. Equal effort for education about psychosocial and peer-delivered care would also be valuable. Partnering with advocacy groups might be a natural step in these regards. As noted above under Element 8, Popular Demand, general efforts to improve (mental) health literacy might be helpful; the public should know about the value of active-engagement treatments in addition to passive ones.

The coupling of Element 2 and 9, pharma/product industry and AMCs respectively, is an issue that is already being debated and partly addressed within pharma as well as in AMCs, through discussions and policy around conflicts of interest, appropriate access of marketing efforts to doctors, and the responsible use of pharma-supported clinical research data. This discussion is likely to go on for some time, as the issues are complicated—we don't want to stifle creativity and new drug treatments, nor do we want to have undue influence of pharma.

As Cosgrove and Krimsky [44] have recently argued, simple disclosure of industry relationships is not sufficient to manage the conflicts of interest manifested in DSM committee service. The problem is complex, because many, perhaps most, recognized experts on this or that disorder have been demonstrated by Cosgrove's group to be highly dependent on industry support. Moreover, temporary divestiture of pharma financial interests during a DSM-development period is more symbolic than substantive in managing the potential for undue influence. Such a skewing of expertise on DSM committees seems likely to skew the nosological vision for past and current DSM efforts, a skewing that favors fewer changes and categories that lend themselves to pharmacological clinical trials and perhaps disorder concepts with more robust marketing potential. So in my view the issue of pharma influence is not just ethical-practical (e.g., bias toward pharma interests), but epistemological (pharma interests influence how DSM committee members think about diagnosis) [4].

This epistemological power of pharma extends, as discussed earlier, not just into DSM committees (Element 10, APA), but also into research study section members (Element 7, NIMH) whose history, funding, and research interests may be unduly DSM-loyal. I should not overlook Element 1 (millions of mentally ill people) and Element 8 (Popular Demand) shaped by advertising, media coverage, and DSM category names which enter into the pop-culture parlance [4, 5]. I believe the issue of conceptual bias described here for the DSMs could be corrected, rather simply, by rethinking the appointments to the DSM Task Forces and Work Groups, and as suggested in the earlier Kendler et al. [82], a more dedicated and direct effort to incorporate the literature on conceptual/philosophical issues into a DSM Work Group which would have actionable input into DSM categories, but also the discussion of diagnostic concepts across broad categories of disorder. I also believe that the divesting of industry funding, at least for the period immediately preceding and following DSM committee work, offers at least a gesture toward a minimally adequate approach to conflict of interest, and may be the wave of the future, if NIH's recent tightening of AMCs' conflict-of-interest rules are an indication [83]. However, as noted earlier, a return to pharma funding outside of DSM activities may well undermine any return to objectivity regarding pharma interests and the DSMs. The definitive solution would be to constitute DSM committees with economically diverse members, and conscientiously correct the over-representation of members who have had any substantive pharma interests over the course of their careers.

Regarding the triumvirate of US politics (Element 5), the US healthcare system (Element 4) and the Service Industry (Element 3), my hopes for reform here are much less optimistic [84]. In the US culture where politics may never have been more polarized and antagonistic, where opportunities for influence-peddling by the most wealthy may be unprecedented, and advertising spending and efforts (Element 6) seem much more important to winning elections than comprehensive policy vision and competence in governing, the outlook is grim for more regulation of the MHMIC, or opening up of opportunity for groups outside of the MHMIC at the Federal or national level. Even more concerning is the seeming preference of the majority of American citizens for 45 million uninsured people rather than some form of adequate health care for them, a problem that has remained unsolved in the United States since its inception. Because NIH (and therefore NIMH) answers directly to Congress, funding priorities there seem to be unlikely to change much until lawmakers decide there is a medical-industrial complex problem, or decide that taxpayers' investment in research in psychiatry is not paying off and decide to reduce funds overall (a terrifying but real possibility).

More optimistically, the potential for universal, regulated health care is still present for the United States, attainable through arduous political steps. One can hope for comprehensive campaign-finance reform as the American people tire of, or even are repelled by, attack ads on television. The growing movement for recovery and patient empowerment, even endorsed by NIMH to some degree [85], could contribute to reform through addressing the aforementioned psychosocial, access to care, conceptual, and patient involvement issues [86].

Regarding the DSM, many possibilities for change are possible. The DSM-5 Task Force promised a manual with big changes when in the early stages of work, but current trends seem to suggest backpedaling on innovations, perhaps in response to outcries of protest [87]. Perhaps NIMH's interest in the RDoC idea signals a new responsiveness to other and more alternatives to the DSM. Perhaps the DSM-5 idea about a "living document" may lead to support for "open source" classifications of disorder, subject to testing and modifications by anyone with a panel of patients who is interested. Only time will tell.

References

1. American Psychiatric Association. Diagnostic and statistical manual of mental disorders. 3rd ed. Washington: American Psychiatric Association; 1980.
2. Wallace ER. Psychiatry and its nosology: a historico-philosophical overview. In: Sadler JZ, Wiggins OP, Schwartz MA, editors. Philosophical perspectives on psychiatric diagnostic classification. Baltimore: The Johns Hopkins University Press; 1994. p. 16–86.
3. Sadler JZ. Descriptions and prescriptions: values, mental disorders, and the DSMs. Baltimore: The Johns Hopkins University Press; 2002.
4. Sadler JZ. Values and psychiatric diagnosis. Oxford/New York: Oxford University Press; 2005.
5. Charland LC. A madness for identity: psychiatric labels, consumer autonomy, and the perils of the Internet. PPP. 2004;11(4):335–49.
6. Schwartz MA, Wiggins OP. The hegemony of the DSMs. In: Sadler JZ, editor. Descriptions and prescriptions: values, mental disorders, and the DSMs. Baltimore: The Johns Hopkins University Press; 2002. p. 199–209.
7. Frances AJ, First MB, Pincus H. DSM-IV guidebook: the essential companion to the diagnostic and statistical manual of mental disorders. 4th ed. Washington: American Psychiatric Association; 1995.
8. World Health Organization. The ICD-10 classification of mental and behavioural disorders: clinical descriptions and diagnostic guidelines. Geneva: World Health Organization; 1992.
9. Sadler JZ, Wiggins OP, Schwartz MA, editors. Philosophical perspectives on psychiatric diagnostic classification. Baltimore: The Johns Hopkins University Press; 1994.
10. Beutler LE, Malik ML, editors. Rethinking the DSM: a psychological perspective. Washington: American Psychological Association; 2002.
11. Horwitz AV. Creating mental illness. Chicago: University of Chicago Press; 2002.
12. Zachar P. Psychological concepts and biological psychiatry: a philosophical analysis. Amsterdam: J. Benjamins; 2000.
13. Jensen PS, Knapp P, Mrazek DA. Toward a new diagnostic system for child psychopathology: moving beyond the DSM. New York: Guilford; 2006.
14. Cooper R. Classifying madness. A philosophical examination of the diagnostic and statistical manual of mental disorders. New York: Springer; 2005.
15. Cooper R. Psychiatry and the philosophy of science. Montreal: McGill-Queen's University Press; 2007.
16. Murphy D. Psychiatry in the scientific image. Cambridge: MIT; 2006.
17. Phillips J, First M. DSM-5 in the homestretch–1. Integrating the coding systems. Psychiatr Times [Internet], March 7. 2012. http://www.psychiatrictimes.com/blog/phillips/content/article/10168/2043461.
18. American Psychiatric Association. Diagnostic and statistical manual of mental disorders. 4th ed. Washington: American Psychiatric Association; 1994.
19. American Psychiatric Association. Diagnostic and statistical manual of mental disorders, fourth edition, text revision (DSM-IV-TR). Washington: American Psychiatric Association; 2000.
20. American Psychological Association Task Force on Descriptive Behavioral Classification. Progress Report; July 1977. (Thanks to Dr. Roger K. Blashfield for this document).
21. Spitzer RL. Nonmedical myths and DSM-III. APA Monitor. 1981 Oct; 3:33.
22. Smith D, Kraft WA. DSM-III: do psychologists really want an alternative? Am Psychol. 1983;38(7):777–85.
23. Tsuang MT, Stone WS, Faraone SV. Toward reformulating the diagnosis of schizophrenia. Am J Psychiatry. 2000;157(7):1041–50.
24. Tsuang MT, Faraone SV, Lyons MJ. Identification of the phenotype in psychiatric genetics. Eur Arch Psychiatry Clin Neurosci. 1993;243(3–4):131–42.
25. Follette WC. Introduction to the special section on the development of theoretically coherent alternatives to the DSM system. J Consult Clin Psychol. 1996;64(6):1117–9.

26. Gottesman II, Gould TD. The endophenotype concept in psychiatry: etymology and strategic intentions. Am J Psychiatry. 2003;160(4):636–45.
27. Walters JT, Owen MJ. Endophenotypes in psychiatric genetics. Mol Psychiatry. 2007; 12(10):886–90.
28. Hyman SE. Can neuroscience be integrated into the DSM-V? Nat Rev Neurosci. 2007; 8:725–32.
29. Hyman SE, Fenton WS. Medicine. What are the right targets for psychopharmacology? Science. 2003;299(5605):350–1.
30. Insel TR, Wang PS. Rethinking mental illness. JAMA. 2010;303(19):1970–1.
31. National Institute of Mental Health. NIMH strategic plan. Bethesda: National Institute of Mental Health; 2008.
32. National Institute of Mental Health. RDoC Draft 3.1 June 2011 [Internet]. June 2011. http://www.nimh.nih.gov/research-funding/rdoc/nimh-research-domain-criteria.
33. Sadler JZ. Psychiatric molecular genetics and the ethics of social promises. J Bioeth Inq. 2011;8:27–34.
34. US Government. Public papers of the Presidents, Dwight D. Eisenhower. [Internet] 1960, p 1035–40. http://quod.lib.umich.edu/p/ppotpus/4728424.1960.001/1090?page=root;rgn=full+text;size=100;view=image. Accessed 2012 June 15.
35. Healy B. 2005. Quotation in US News & World Report [Internet]. 2005. http://health.usnews.com/usnews/health/articles/050124/24healy. Accessed 2012 June 15.
36. Kovel J. The American mental health industry. In: Ingleby D, editor. Critical psychiatry: the politics of mental health. New York: Pantheon; 1980. p. 72–101.
37. Sadler JZ, Jotterand F, Lee SC, Inrig S. Can medicalization be good? Situating medicalization within bioethics. Theor Med Bioeth. 2009;30:411–25.
38. Phillips J, editor. Philosophical perspectives on technology and psychiatry. Oxford: Oxford University Press; 2009.
39. Pincus H, Frances A, Davis WW, First M, Widiger T. DSM-IV and new diagnostic categories: holding the line on proliferation. Am J Psychiatry. 1992;149(1):112–7.
40. Lane C. Shyness: how normal behavior became a sickness. New Haven: Yale University Press; 2008.
41. Horwitz AV, Wakefield JC. The loss of sadness: how psychiatry transformed normal sorrow into depressive disorder. New York/Oxford: Oxford University Press; 2007.
42. Cosgrove L, Krimsky S, Vijayaraghavan M, Schneider L. Financial ties between DSM-IV panel members and the pharmaceutical industry. Psychother Psychosom. 2006;75:154–60.
43. Cosgrove L, Bursztajn HJ, Krimsky S, Anaya M, Walker J. Conflicts of interest and disclosure in the American Psychiatric Association's Clinical Practice Guidelines. Psychother Psychosom. 2009;78:228–32.
44. Cosgrove L, Krimsky S. A comparison of DSM-IV and DSM-5 panel members financial associations with industry: a pernicious problem persists. PLoS Med. 2009;9(3):e1001190.
45. Parens E, Johnston J. Troubled children: diagnosing, treating, and attending to context. Special report. Hastings Cent Rep. 2011;41(2):S1–32.
46. Blendon RJ, Benson JM. Americans' views on health policy: a fifty-year historical perspective. Health Aff. 2001;20(2):33–46.
47. Iglehart JK. Health policy report: the American health care system: medicare. N Engl J Med. 1992;327:1467–72.
48. Iglehart JK. Rallying the caucus—The Democrats struggle for unity on reform. N Engl J Med. 2009;361:e64.
49. Sparer M. Medicaid and the U.S. path to national health insurance. N Engl J Med. 2009;360:323–5.
50. De Tocqueville A. Democracy in America [H. C. Mansfield, D. Winthrop, trans]. Chicago: University of Chicago Press; 2000.
51. Bellah RN, Madsen R, Sullivan WM, Swidler A, Tipton SM. Habits of the heart: individualism and commitment in American life. Berkeley: University of California Press; 2008.
52. Landers SH, Sehgal AR. Health care lobbying in the United States. Am J Med. 2004;116(7):474–7.

53. Abraham J. The pharmaceutical industry as a political player. Lancet. 2002;360(9344):1498–502.
54. Citizens United v. Federal Election Commission. 558 U.S. Supreme Court (201). Opinion of Stevens, J.
55. Harris G. Drug makers are advocacy groups biggest donors. The New York Times 2009 Oct 21.
56. NAMI. Major foundation and corporate support [Internet]. http://www.nami.org/Content/ NavigationMenu/Inform_Yourself/About_NAMI/Governance/Major_Foundation_and_ Corporate_Support/NAMI_Corporate_Relations_and_Giving_Policies.htm.
57. Mental Health America. 2010 Annual report. Alexandria: MHA; 2010.
58. Donohue JM, Cevasco M, Rosenthal MB. A decade of direct-to-consumer advertising of prescription drugs. N Engl J Med. 2007;357:673–81.
59. Potter W. Deadly spin: an insurance company insider speaks out on how corporate PR is killing health care and deceiving Americans. New York: Bloomsbury; 2009.
60. Grob GN. The mad among us: a history of the care of America's mentally ill. New York: Free Press; 1994.
61. Healy D. The creation of psychopharmacology. Cambridge: Harvard University Press; 2002.
62. Healy D. Let them eat prozac: the unhealthy relationship between the pharmaceutical industry and depression. New York: NYU; 2004.
63. Dwan K, Altman DG, Arnaiz JA, Bloom J, Chan A-W, Cronin E, et al. Systematic review of the empirical evidence of study publication bias and outcome reporting bias. PLoS One. 2008;3(8):e3081. doi:doi: 10.1371/journal.pone.0003081.
64. Ghaemi SN. The failure to know what isn't known: negative publication bias with lamotrigine and a glimpse inside peer review. Evid Based Ment Health. 2009;12:65–8.
65. Turner EH, Matthews AM, Linardatos E, Tell RA, Rosenthal R. Selective publication of antidepressant trials and its influence on apparent efficacy. N Engl J Med. 2008;358:252–60.
66. Zimmerman M. Why are we rushing to publish DSM-IV? Arch Gen Psychiatry. 1988;45(12):1135–8.
67. Zimmerman M. Is DSM-IV needed at all? Arch Gen Psychiatry. 1990;47(10):974–6.
68. Devisch I. Co-responsibility: a new horizon for today's health care? Health Care Anal. 2012;20:139–51.
69. Jones GK, Brewer KL, Garrison HG. Public expectations of survival following cardiopulmonary resuscitation. Acad Emerg Med. 2000;7(1):48–53.
70. Rosenberg CE. Disease and social order in America: perceptions and expectations. Milbank Q. 1986;64 Suppl 1:34–55.
71. Scott TL, Gazmararian JA, Williams MV, Baker DW. Health literacy and preventive health care use among medicare enrollees in a managed care organization. Med Care. 2002;40(5):395–404.
72. Shieh C, Halstead JA. Understanding the impact of health literacy on women's health. J Obstet Gynecol Neonatal Nurs. 2009;38(5):601–10.
73. Williams MV, Davis T, Parker RM, Weiss BD. The role of health literacy in patient-physician communication. Fam Med. 2002;34(5):383–9.
74. Sadler JZ. The instrument metaphor, hyponarrativity, and the generic clinician. In: Phillips J, editor. Philosophical perspectives on technology and psychiatry. Oxford: Oxford University Press; 2009. p. 23–33.
75. Light DW. Toward a new sociology of medical education. J Health Soc Behav. 1988;29:307–22.
76. Starr P. The social transformation of American medicine. The rise of a sovereign profession and the making of a vast industry. New York: Basic Books; 1982.
77. Rothman D, editor. Combating conflict of interest: a primer for countering industry marketing. New York: Institute on Medicine as a Profession; 2012.
78. Guyatt G et al. Evidence based medicine: a new approach to teaching the practice of medicine. J Am Med Assoc. 1992;268(17):2420–5.
79. Sackett DL, Rosenberg WMC, Muir Gray JA, Haynes RB, Richardson WS. Evidence based medicine: what it is and what it isn't. BMJ. 1996;312:71.

80. Gupta M. Does evidence based medicine apply to psychiatry? Theor Med Bioeth. 2007; 28:103–20.
81. Blashfield R. Taxonomy of psychopathology blog [Internet]. http://taxonpsych.blogspot.com/.
82. Kendler KS, Appelbaum PS, Bell CC, Fulford KWM, Ghaemi SN, Schaffner KF, et al. Editorial: Issues for DSM-V: DSM-V should include a conceptual issues work group. Am J Psychiatry. 2008;165(2):174–5.
83. National Institutes of Health. HHS tightens financial conflict of interest rules for researchers [Internet]. 2011. http://www.nih.gov/news/health/aug2011/od-23.htm.
84. Relman AS. A second opinion: rescuing America's health care. New York: Public Affairs; 2007.
85. National Advisory Mental Health Council's Workgroup. From discovery to cure: accelerating the development of new and personalized interventions for mental illnesses. Bethesda: National Institute of Mental Health; 2010.
86. Sadler JZ, Fulford KWM. Should patients and families contribute to the DSM-V process? Psychiatr Serv. 2004;55(2):133–8.
87. Frances A. Wonderful news: DSM-5 finally begins its belated and necessary retreat. Psychiatr Times [Internet]. 2012 [2012 May 4]. http://www.psychiatrictimes.com/blog/frances/content/article/10168/2068571.

Chapter 3
The Ideology Behind DSM-5

Joel Paris

Ideology and Neuroscience

An ideology provides a comprehensive vision. The problem is that ideological thinking may not correspond to the complexities and inconsistencies of the real world. That is obvious in politics, but the principle also applies to science. While scientists do not believe that they think ideologically, they often pretend to know more than they do. For this reason, theories that seem to explain everything can take on the cast of belief. Yet paradigms can be overthrown, and the most powerful theories have been undermined by new facts [1].

Medicine is a practical discipline. A classification of disease is primarily intended for communication, and is usually provisional. The mechanisms of only a few diseases are understood well enough for diagnosis to be firmly based on science. Diagnostic systems are particularly bound to be messy in psychiatry, a field that concerns the vast complexities of mind and brain.

Faced with this daunting challenge, most psychiatrists have often been humble. Emil Kraepelin [2], rejecting the world-embracing but speculative ideology of psychoanalysis, argued that until more was known about the brain, psychiatry had no choice but to await further discoveries, and, in the meantime, to focus on a precise description of psychopathology. This "phenomenological" tradition came to dominate European psychiatry and was revived in the USA as a "neo-Kraepelinian" school [3]. Beginning in 1980, this point of view, in which clinical phenomena are reliably observed while etiological speculations are viewed with caution, has been central to the DSM system.

J. Paris (✉)
Jewish General Hospital, Department of Psychiatry, McGill University,
4333 Cote Ste. Catherine, Montreal, QC, Canada, H3T1E4
e-mail: joel.paris@mcgill.ca

J. Paris and J. Phillips (eds.), *Making the DSM-5: Concepts and Controversies*,
DOI 10.1007/978-1-4614-6504-1_3, © Springer Science+Business Media New York 2013

Over the last quarter century, some mysteries of the brain have begun to be illuminated by researches using new technologies. The advance of neuroscience led to the hope that mental disorders could be explained through genetics, neuro-chemistry, neuro-circuitry, and neuroimaging. Psychiatry as a whole has adopted this point of view, and some proponents have even suggested that psychiatry should rejoin neurology, and redefine itself as the clinical application of neuro-science [4].

This point of view runs contrary to the long influential principle that psychiatry requires a biopsychosocial model [5]. Rejecting these traditional roots, neuroscience-based psychiatry is firmly reductionistic, viewing mind as an epiphenomenon of brain. Unfortunately biological reductionism fails to acknowledge that complex systems have emergent properties that cannot entirely be explained on the basis of components [6]. While mind cannot exist without brain, it cannot be fully reduced to neuro-circuitry or cellular mechanisms.

Given the dominance of the neuroscience ideology over the last 20 years, it is not surprising that the DSM-5 process was put in the hands of those who believe in it. The editors of the new edition [7] make it clear that psychiatric diagnosis should be based on neuroscience. While they acknowledge that this line of research has not yet explained the cause of any mental disorder, they propose broad spectra of psy-chopathology that might be closer to biological markers than traditional diagnostic categories. This idea has also been taken up by the National Institute of Mental Health (NIMH) [8], which proposes that all future research should be based on these spectra, defined as Research Domain Criteria (RDoCs).

Yet no mental disorder is associated with a consistent biological marker, either from neurochemistry or from imaging data. This suggests that psychopathology is too complex to be readily classified, either in distinct categories, or in broad spectra. For example, the fact that psychopharmacological agents change brain chemistry does not prove that mental disorders are caused by "chemical imbalances." Similarly, the fact that mental disorders are associated with changes in brain function that can be measured by imaging does not prove that alterations in the activity of neuro-circuitry are the cause of these illnesses. It could be decades before we understand the brain well enough to apply that knowledge to practice. Finally, all currently defined "dimensions" or "spectra" of psychopathology are based entirely on clinical observation. Clinical rating scales or self-report measures can provide greater precision of observation, but they are not independent measures like blood pressure or an electrocardiogram.

Given the limited state of evidence in support of spectra, the adoption of RDoCs by NIMH can only be described as ideological. Putting the problem in a broader scientific perspective, the brain is the most complex structure in the entire universe. It is therefore not surprising that neuroscience is in its infancy. Rushing ahead to doubtfully valid spectra that are not yet rooted in data shows a lack of patience and a lack of judgment. While no one can deny dramatic progress in neuroscience, this research has not yet had any direct application to psychiatry. We still do not know whether most conditions listed in the diagnostic manual are true diseases. We are no closer to understanding the etiology and pathogenesis of mental disorders than 50 years ago. For this reason, DSM-5 had no choice but to continue with a provisional and pragmatic classification system based on phenomenological observation. The establishment of biological mechanisms and markers remains a long-term goal. But DSM-5 has been written for 2013, not for 2063 or 2113.

Why DSM-5 Adopted Its Ideology

What lies behind the ideology of DSM-5? Psychiatry has long been notably different from all other fields of medicine. In the past, practitioners spent long hours talking to people about their lives. Prescriptions were written with caution. But psychiatrists got little respect for conducting a humanistic practice. Medical colleagues sometimes treated the specialty with contempt. And research psychologists pointed out the unreliability of the observational data on which diagnosis was based.

In a kind of "internist envy," psychiatrists wanted to be seen in the same way as every other specialty. Diagnosing and treating mental illness on the basis of neuroscience aimed to provide the field with legitimacy [9, 10]. While one can understand the motives behind this position, it does not change the fact that theories of mental illness are well behind the rest of medicine. Psychiatry is still waiting for its Pasteur, Koch, or Virchow. When it comes to treatment, our effectiveness can be at least as good as what medical colleagues have to offer [11]. Yet psychiatric diagnosis remains syndromal, a rough-and-ready system that communicates but rarely explains.

Psychopathology and Normality

Another ideological element in DSM-5 is that there is no essential difference between normality and psychopathology. The conviction that mental disorder is a point on a continuum follows directly from a neuroscience-based dimensional model. It is true that research has failed to establish any precise distinction between mental illness and normality, and that the few biological markers we have are more associated with traits than with categories of disorder. But while categories of illness, whether in medicine or psychiatry, are often fuzzy around the edges, it does not follow that we should discard them. The danger of the DSM-5 ideology is that it extends the scope of mental disorder to a point where almost anyone can be diagnosed with one (and treated accordingly).

The principle that there is a fundamental difference between pathology and normality goes back to Kraepelin, and was hard fought for by the editors of DSM-III. It was opposed by psychoanalysts explained all human thought, emotion, and behavior using one theory. Now in the name of neuroscience, we are in danger of returning to these bad old days. Admittedly, there can never be a sharp distinction between illness and life. However, differences in degree can also be differences in kind.

Let us consider some examples of dangers associated with broader spectra and broader diagnoses. Let us begin with depression. The current definition of "major depression" is very broad, crossing the boundary to normal variation. It confuses mental disorder with normal unhappiness and grief [12]. That is why up to half the population can meet criteria for major depression over a lifetime [13]. One important result of this confusion is that psychiatrists are treating unhappiness with drugs. That goes a long way to explaining why 11 % of the adult population is on an antidepressant [14].

A second example is anxiety disorders. Overly broad definitions in the DSM manual of generalized anxiety disorder and posttraumatic stress disorder fail to separate pathological and irrational symptoms to reactions to real dangers [15]. And the broader a diagnostic concept, the more treatment takes place. This confusion has been another reason for the ubiquity of antidepressant drugs.

A third example is the (now-shelved) proposal to diagnose patients with subclinical symptoms resembling schizophrenia with an "attenuated psychosis syndrome" [16]. Again, based on the principle that subthreshold presentations are milder forms of classical disorders, attenuated symptoms would be treated in the same way. In the end, the reason for shelving the proposal was that it would have led to unnecessary treatment for about 70 % of these cases, which never develop into schizophrenia [17].

A fourth example is the bipolar spectrum. This idea suggests that mood instability, both in clinical populations and in the population at large, should be diagnosed as a variant of bipolar disorder [18]. The spectrum has been promoted by claims [19] that up to 40 % of all outpatients suffer from a form of bipolarity. Thus, even though DSM-5 has not reduced the requirements for a hypomanic episode, clinicians have been encouraged to diagnose bipolarity in patients with mood swings [20]. One epidemiological study [21] that examined subclinical moodiness in community populations went so far as to express concern that people with subclinical symptoms are not being "treated." Needless to say, these conclusions would lead to an even more striking increase in the prescription rate for mood stabilizers and atypical antipsychotics.

A fifth example is autism. The concept of autistic spectrum disorder is broad, and not restricted to the classic clinical picture [22]. Interpreted liberally, it might absorb all eccentrics on the planet. One epidemiological survey [23] has claimed community rates as high as 4 % for what used to be considered a rare disorder. While there is no pharmacological treatment for autism, but overidentification could have other hazards, such as stigmatization.

A sixth example is attention-deficit hyperactivity disorder (ADHD). Since its boundaries with normal variations in attention are by no means clear, there has been a diagnostic epidemic in recent years, particularly in adults [24].

A seventh example is personality disorder. This diagnosis can be unpopular, in part because it points to treatment with psychotherapy rather than with drugs. While a radical proposal to revised the personality disorder section was rejected in December, 2012, the definitions in DSM-5 do not define a clear border between personality disorder and normal personality. As with most disorders in DSM, diagnostic criteria have been loose, resulting in a community prevalence of 10 % or more [25]. While it is credible that one out of ten of us have problems managing interpersonal relations and occupational tasks, such difficulties fall within the range of normality, and need not define a mental disorder. Moreover, overdiagnosis trivializes the serious clinical challenges of severe personality disorder.

A final example is substance abuse. The decision of DSM-5 to call all such cases "addiction" is in accord with a general tendency to see everything as lying on a continuum, with disorder defined by severity. In this case, the absence of a boundary between pathology and normality means that at least 10 % of the population can receive a diagnosis [26].

All these examples demonstrate the practical consequences of applying the DSM-5 ideology. The lifetime prevalence of mental disorder will be close to 100 %. More and more people will receive treatment, whether they need it or not. And most of this treatment will consist of pharmacological interventions.

Ideology and Hubris

The ideology of DSM-5 exaggerates what we know, and reflects impatience for a time when psychiatrists can practice in the same way other physicians. However, it is doubtful whether changes of this extent in theory and practice are, as we are often told, "just around the corner." The claim that we can apply neuroscience to diagnosis, creating valid spectra of psychopathology, is little but hubris.

Moreover, the DSM-5 approach supports some of the most problematic aspects of current practice. Although every manual since DSM-III has included a warning not to use the text as a guide to treatment, clinicians have paid little attention. It is too tempting to make a quick diagnosis and pull out a prescription pad.

With time, neuroscience will eventually enrich psychiatry, and help it manage severely ill patients. However much of psychiatric and primary care practice still focus on "common mental disorders" such as depression and anxiety, as well as addictions and personality disorders. These problems do not have an easy psychopharmacological solution, and there is still an important role for talking to patients, even if psychiatrists are doing so less and less of that. The concepts promoted by the DSM-5 ideology do not contradict taking the time to get a life history, but its focus on symptom checklists certainly does not encourage it.

References

1. Kuhn TA. The structure of scientific revolutions. 2nd ed. Chicago: University of Chicago Press; 1970.
2. Kraepelin, E. Manic-depressive insanity and paranoia (R. M. Barclay, Trans.). Robertson GM, editor. Edinburgh: E & S Livingstone; 1921.
3. Klerman G. Historical perspectives on contemporary schools of psychopathology. In: Millon T, Klerman G, editors. Contemporary psychopathology: towards the DSM-IV. New York: Guilford; 1986. p. 3–28.

4. Insel T, Quirion R. Psychiatry as a clinical neuroscience discipline. JAMA. 2005;294:2221–4.
5. Engel GL. The clinical application of the biopsychosocial model. Am J Psychiatry. 1980; 137:535–44.
6. Gold I. Reduction in psychiatry. Can J Psychiatry. 2009;54:506–12.
7. Kupfer DJ, Regier DA. Neuroscience, clinical evidence, and the future of psychiatric classification in DSM-5. Am J Psychiatry. 2011;168:172–4.
8. Insel TR. A strategic plan for research on mental illness: translating scientific opportunity into public health impact. Arch Gen Psychiatry. 2009;66:128–33.
9. Carlat D. Unhinged. New York: Free Press; 2010.
10. Paris J. Prescriptions for the mind. New York: Oxford University Press; 2008.
11. Leucht S, Hierl S, Kissling W, Dold M, Davis JM. Putting the efficacy of psychiatric and general medicine medication into perspective: review of meta-analyses. Br J Psychiatry. 2012; 200:97–106.
12. Horwitz AV, Wakefield JC. The loss of sadness: how psychiatry transformed normal sorrow into depressive disorder. New York: Oxford University Press; 2007.
13. Moffitt TE, Caspi A, Taylor A, Kokaua J. How common are common mental disorders? Evidence that lifetime prevalence rates are doubled by prospective versus retrospective ascertainment. Psychol Med. 2009;940:899–909.
14. Pratt LA, Brody DJ, Gu Q. Antidepressant use in persons aged 12 and over: United States, 2005–2008. NCHS data brief, no 76. Hyattsville, MD: National Center for Health Statistics; 2011.
15. Horwitz AV, Wakefield JC. All we have to fear: psychiatry's transformation of natural anxieties into mental disorders. New York: Oxford University Press; 2012.
16. Carpenter WT. Anticipating DSM-V: should psychosis risk become a diagnostic class? Schizophr Bull. 2009;35:841–3.
17. Cannon TD, Cadenhead K, Cornblatt B, Woods SW, Addington J, Walker E, et al. Prediction of psychosis in youth at high clinical risk: a multisite longitudinal study in North America. Arch Gen Psychiatry. 2008;65:28–37.
18. Akiskal HS. The bipolar spectrum: the shaping of a new paradigm in psychiatry. Curr Psychiatry Rep. 2002;4:1–3.
19. Angst J, Gamma A. A new bipolar spectrum concept: a brief review. Bipolar Disord. 2002; 4:11–4.
20. Merikangas KR, Akiskal HS, Angst J, Greenberg PE, Hirschfeld RM, Petukhova M, et al. Lifetime and 12-month prevalence of bipolar spectrum disorder in the National Comorbidity Survey Replication. Arch Gen Psychiatry. 2007;64:543–52.
21. Paris J. The bipolar spectrum—diagnosis or fad? New York: Routledge; 2012.
22. Brugha TS, McManus S, Bankart J. Epidemiology of autism spectrum disorders in adults in the community in England. Arch Gen Psychiatry. 2011;68:459–65.
23. Kim YS, Leventhal BL, Koh Y-J, Fombonne E, Laska E, Lim EC, et al. Prevalence of autism spectrum disorders in a total population sample. Am J Psychiatry. 2011;168(9):904–12.
24. Batstra L, Frances AJ. DSM-5 further inflates attention deficit hyperactivity disorder. J Nerv Ment Dis. 2012;200:486–8.
25. Paris J. Estimating the prevalence of personality disorders. J Pers Disord. 2010;24:405–11.
26. Frances, A. DSM-5: "Addiction" swallows substance abuse. Psychiatric Times. March 30, 2010.

Part II
Ideological *and* Conceptual Perspectives

Chapter 4
The Biopolitics of Defining "Mental Disorder"

Warren Kinghorn

What is psychiatry, and how does it relate to other medical and mental health disciplines? Apart from the obvious sociological answer—psychiatrists are physicians who have completed residency training in psychiatry—psychiatry has always struggled to define itself with precision. Unlike pediatrics or geriatrics, psychiatry does not define itself by reference to a specific demographic population. Unlike general surgery or anesthesiology or radiology, it does not define itself exclusively with reference to specific technologies or interventional practices: the majority of psychotropic medications in the United States are prescribed by nonpsychiatrists [1]. Unlike certain medical specialties such as nephrology or cardiology, psychiatry cannot lay exclusive claim to a particular body part or organ system: although psychiatry is often referred to as a "clinical neuroscience" [2], psychiatry at best shares this distinction with neurology, neurosurgery, and neuropsychology. Nor can psychiatry define itself according to a particular institutional structure of practice, since psychiatrists have long shed their historic identification with inpatient institutions and now work within a broad and diverse array of practice settings.

Lacking any more salient identifier, American psychiatry has most consistently defined itself according to the conditions which it treats: a psychiatrist, as the American Psychiatric Association (APA) presently states on its public website, is "a medical doctor who specializes in the diagnosis, treatment and prevention of mental health, including substance use disorders" [3]. Psychiatrists, in other words, are clinicians who (unlike psychologists, social workers, and other therapists) are "medical doctors" and who (unlike other physicians) focus on certain things called "mental disorders." The concept of "mental disorder," then, plays an important role in the way that psychiatry publicly describes itself as a distinct and coherent medical specialty.

W. Kinghorn, MD, ThD (✉)
Department of Psychiatry and Behavioral Sciences, Duke University Medical Center
and Duke Divinity School, Box 90968, Duke Divinity School, Durham, NC 27708, USA
e-mail: warren.kinghorn@duke.edu

J. Paris and J. Phillips (eds.), *Making the DSM-5: Concepts and Controversies*, 47
DOI 10.1007/978-1-4614-6504-1_4, © Springer Science+Business Media New York 2013

   The problem with publicly defining itself in this way is that psychiatry has never been able to settle on a precise and unambiguous conceptual description of "mental disorder." Most of the time, to be sure, this hasn't mattered very much for everyday psychiatric practice: patients come to psychiatrists not because they care about the precise meaning of "mental disorder" but because they want to feel, think, or act better. In this light, specific behavioral, cognitive, and emotional configurations such as schizophrenia, bipolar disorder, and panic disorder are generally accepted as mental disorders which are appropriate objects of psychiatric evaluation and treatment. But in moments when psychiatry's authority or helpfulness has been questioned, the concept of "mental disorder" becomes much more visible and important. At these times—notably in the case of homosexuality [4] but also in the cases of social phobia [5], major depressive disorder [6], certain of the paraphilias [7], and other disorders—critics of the *DSM* often frame their criticism by questioning whether the pathologized experience or behavior is in fact appropriately described as "mental illness" or "mental disorder." Indeed, a large theme of the so-called antipsychiatry movement of the past 50 years has been that "mental disorder" is itself a circular concept, that psychiatry attains and asserts its power and influence by colonizing particular domains of human life and culture as "mental illnesses" and then by offering itself as the appropriate authority for their "treatment" [5, 8, 9]. In these cases, critics argue, a psychiatric profession which defines itself as the medical discipline which treats "mental disorders" ought to be able to define "mental disorders" as something other than "the conditions which psychiatrists treat."

   In the context of such public questioning of psychiatry and the need to position psychiatry as a medical discipline distinct from other medical disciplines, philosophers, psychiatrists, and other mental health professionals over the past four decades have devoted much time, effort, and energy toward the development of a precise, consensual, noncircular definition of mental disorder—a quest which persists to this day in *DSM-5*. In this chapter, I will argue that this quest has little to do with the scientific and pragmatic utility of such a definition—which has historically been nearly irrelevant and in the future is likely to be modest at best—and much to do with the political force of a clear definition. I will argue that the project to define "mental disorder" arose in the 1970s and early 1980s as a way to burnish the authority of psychiatry and specifically of *DSM-III*. I will argue that the project to define "mental disorder" has continued in subsequent editions of *DSM,* including *DSM-5,* primarily in order to persuade internal and external constituents that there exists an appropriate, safe, and nonthreatening clinical "space" within which psychiatric diagnosis and treatment can be rightfully exercised. But I will conclude by arguing that there is no such safe space for psychiatry and that the *DSM* definition of "mental disorder" ought therefore to be discarded.

A Political History of the *DSM* Definition of "Mental Disorder"

Although speculation about the nature of mental illness had ample precedent within psychiatry, the modern *DSM* definition of mental disorder traces its roots to the 1970s as American psychiatry confronted a scientific and social "crisis of legitimacy" [10].

Social trust in psychiatrists' ability to speak authoritatively about human life and suffering was challenged by the countercultural and antiauthoritarian movements of the 1960s and 1970s; these challenges were displayed in specific events such as Thomas Szasz' publication of *The Myth of Mental Illness* [8], Erving Goffman's expose and critique of psychiatric institutions [11], the commercial success and cinematographic portrayal of Ken Kesey's *One Flew Over the Cuckoo's Nest* [12], the publication in *Science* of the so-called Rosenhan experiments in which a group of researchers feigned psychosis in order to gain access to psychiatric hospitals and then were able to gain release only after lengthy admissions [13], and perhaps most notably, the protracted debate within the APA which led to the removal of homosexuality from *DSM-II* in 1973 [4]. In response to these external and internal challenges to psychiatry's authority and legitimacy, empirically minded research psychiatrists began to advocate that psychiatry more closely attend to its status as a modern biomedical discipline: the psychiatry that they envisioned would be less politically engaged and psychoanalytically oriented and more oriented toward traditional medical models of disease, diagnosis, and treatment. The groundbreaking work of the APA Task Force on Nomenclature and Statistics which culminated in the publication of *DSM-III* in 1980 was both the fruit and a catalyst of this movement: with its ostensive commitment to construct reliability and etiological theory-neutrality, *DSM-III* embodied its creators' hope for a psychiatry which was "[reliant] on data as the basis for understanding mental disorders" [14].

In the context of this larger effort to shore up the philosophical and medical legitimacy of psychiatry and to ward off sociopolitical critique of the profession, psychiatrists (along with other physicians) began to think and write more about the concept of disease and, specifically, the concept of "mental illness" or "mental disorder." R. E. Kendell, for instance, while conceding that the concept of disease was unnecessary for most psychiatric practice and that medicine had never organized its nosology around a unified concept of disease, cited the anti-psychiatry movement as justification for the need for a definition of mental illness and modified a prior definition of J. G. Scadding [15] to describe disease as a deviation from a species norm which results in increased mortality or decreased fertility [16]. Donald Klein defined disease as "covert, objective, suboptimal part dysfunction"— linking disease to the loss of "optimal biological functioning, within an evolutionary context"—and defined mental illness as "the subset of all illness that presents evidence in the cognitive, behavioral, affective, and motivational aspects of organismic functioning" [17].

The *DSM* definition of mental disorder emerged in the context of these clinical and philosophical conversations and owes its existence primarily to Robert Spitzer, the chair of the APA Task Force on Nomenclature and Statistics and the principal architect of *DSM-III*. Spitzer had been involved in the *DSM-II* revision process but had gained further stature and visibility within American psychiatry through his politically deft actions to resolve the controversy over the diagnostic status of homosexuality in *DSM-II*. Mindful of the mounting political cost of psychiatry's pathologization of homosexuality and personally sympathetic to the arguments and claims of psychiatrists who described themselves as gay, Spitzer navigated a 1973 compromise in which homosexuality per se would be removed from *DSM-II* but a residual category, Sexual Orientation Disorder, would remain. Writing later of this process, Spitzer stated that his evolving attitudes regarding homosexuality had been guided by a conviction that mental illnesses either "regularly caused subjective distress or were associated with generalized impairment in social effectiveness or functioning," neither of which applied to homosexuality per se [18]. Spitzer and Jean Endicott (1978) stated that the homosexuality controversy provided the "initial impetus" for the effort to place a definition of mental disorder in *DSM-III*. (Neither *DSM-I* nor *DSM-II* had included any such definition.) They stated that the conviction that a definition was needed grew as the *DSM-III* revision process began in 1975:

> Decisions had to be made on a variety of issues that seemed to relate to the fundamental question of the boundaries of the concept of mental disorder. We believed that without some definition of mental disorder, there would be no explicit guiding principles that would help to determine which conditions should be included in the nomenclature, which excluded, and how included conditions should be defined [19].

Spitzer and Endicott proposed a draft definition of mental disorder at the 1976 APA annual meeting and found that "to our chagrin, the reaction was negative" [19]. Respondents and audience members charged that a definition of mental disorder was unnecessary, that it would unduly restrict the scope of psychiatric practice, and that it would not be effective in guiding decisions about nomenclature. Undeterred, Spitzer and Endicott revised this draft definition and in 1978 proposed a definition of "mental disorder" as a subset of "medical disorder:"

> A medical disorder is a relatively distinct condition resulting from organismic dysfunction which in its fully developed or extreme form is directly and intrinsically associated with distress, disability, or certain other types of disadvantage. The disadvantage may be of a physical, perceptual, sexual, or interpersonal nature. Implicitly there is a call for action on the part of the person who has the condition, the medical or its allied professions, and society. A mental disorder is a medical disorder whose manifestations are primarily signs or symptoms of a psychological (behavioral) nature, or if physical, can be understood only using psychological concepts [19].

Spitzer and Williams report that this definition, too, was received tepidly by the APA Task Force on Nomenclature and Statistics. In addition to this, the American Psychological Association strongly dissented to any concept of "mental disorder" as a subset of "medical disorder" [20, 21]. They write that after an "agonizing _ reappraisal," the Task Force decided to eliminate any referent to "medical disorder" from the *DSM* definition. They report that work on the definition then stopped for several years until "eventually, in the last few months of work on *DSM-III* another attempt was made to define mental disorder incorporating certain key concepts that had been helpful in providing a rationale for decisions as to which conditions should be included or excluded from the *DSM-III* classification of mental disorders and as guides in defining the boundaries of the various mental disorders" [20]. This revised definition appeared in *DSM-III*, following the qualifying statement that "there is no satisfactory definition that specifies precise boundaries for the concept 'mental disorder' (also true for such concepts as physical disorder and mental and physical health)," as follows:

In *DSM-III* each of the mental disorders is conceptualized as a clinically significant behavioral or psychological syndrome or pattern that occurs in an individual and that is typically associated with either a painful symptom (distress) or impairment in one or more important areas of functioning (disability). In addition, there is an inference that there is a behavioral, psychological, or biological dysfunction, and that the disturbance is not only in the relationship between the individual and society (When the disturbance is *limited* to a conflict between an individual and society, this may represent social deviance, which may or may not be commendable, but is not by itself a mental disorder.) [14].

This definition by Spitzer and colleagues established the basic definitional form which has appeared in each subsequent edition of the *DSM. DSM-III-R* (1987), also edited by Spitzer, revised the definition slightly, adding to "distress" and "disability" the possibility that a person with mental disorder might be at "significantly increased risk of suffering death, pain, disability, or an important loss of freedom. In addition, this syndrome or pattern must not be merely an expectable response to a particular event, e.g., the death of a loved one" [22]. The definition of mental disorder which appears in *DSM-IV* and *DSM-IV-TR,* principally edited by Allen Frances, slightly tweaks the *DSM-III-R* definition without changing it substantially. After a lengthy prefatory comment that as with medical conditions in general, "the concept of mental disorder, like many other concepts in medicine and science, lacks a consistent operational definition which covers all situations," the *DSM-IV* authors state that the *DSM-III-R* definition is being included in *DSM-IV* "because it is as useful as any other available definition and has helped to guide decisions regarding which conditions on the boundary between normality and pathology should be included in *DSM-IV*" [23]. The full *DSM-IV* definition reads as follows:

In DSM-IV, each of the mental disorders is conceptualized as a clinically significant behavioral or psychological syndrome or pattern that occurs in an individual and that is associated with present distress (e.g., a painful symptom) or disability (i.e., impairment in one or more important areas of functioning) or with a significantly increased risk of suffering death, pain, disability, or an important loss of freedom. In addition, this syndrome or pattern must not be merely an expectable and culturally sanctioned response to a particular event, for example, the death of a loved one. Whatever its original cause, it must currently be considered a manifestation of a behavioral, psychological, or biological dysfunction in the individual. Neither deviant behavior (e.g., political, religious, or sexual) nor conflicts that are primarily between the individual and society are mental disorders unless the deviance or conflict is a symptom of a dysfunction in the individual, as described above [23].

Despite Frances' avowal around the time of the *DSM-IV* revision process (and in the text of *DSM-IV* itself) that the *DSM-III-R* definition had played some role in the construction of the *DSM-IV* classification, there is little specific evidence of this. Indeed, even at the time of the *DSM-IV* revision process, Frances and colleagues wrote that "the implicit definition of mental disorders and medical disorders—'that which clinicians treat'—is tautological, but other more abstract concepts consistently fail to provide greater explanatory power" [24].

Although the *DSM-5* definition of mental disorder is still being constructed at the time of this writing, it is expected to take the same general form as the *DSM-III* and *DSM-IV* definitions. The final pre-publication draft definition refers to mental disorders as "health conditions" characterized by "dysfunction in an individual's cognitions, emotions, or behaviors that reflects a disturbance in the psychological, biological, or developmental processes underlying mental functioning." Some disorders, however, "may not be diagnosable until they have caused clinically significant distress or impairment of performance." As in *DSM-IV,* a mental disorder cannot be an expected or culturally sanctioned response to a particular life event and cannot be primarily a conflict between the individual and society, "unless the deviance or conflict results from a dysfunction in the individual" [25].

DSM-5 and the Lure of a Definition

I referred to the previous section as a "political history" of mental disorder definitions to make clear that the *DSM* definition of mental disorder, like the *DSM* itself, did not develop in a historical vacuum; it emerged, rather, at a specific period of psychiatry's history, in response to particular historical events and political challenges, to serve particular functions with regard to psychiatry's relationship to the rest of medicine and to its various constituent groups. Robert Spitzer's extensive engagement in the debate about the diagnostic status of homosexuality forced him (and others) to think critically about the appropriate boundaries of psychiatric diagnosis and convinced him (and some, though not all, others) that a clear definition of "mental disorder" could guide diagnostic decisions in the *DSM-III* revision process. The clear implication of Spitzer's advocacy of a definition of mental disorder was that with the benefit of a well-constructed definition, psychiatry would be less likely to stumble into the politically complicated nosological terrain that had engulfed it in the case of homosexuality.

Despite Spitzer's hope and despite his eventual success in placing a definition of mental disorder in *DSM-III,* it is clear that the *DSM* definition of mental disorder has never played a major role in the revision processes of any edition of the *DSM,* from *DSM-III* to *DSM-5.* Spitzer and Williams (1982) acknowledged this, writing that the *DSM-III* definition of mental disorder was written *after* the major nosological decisions had been made and which at best "[incorporated] certain key concepts that had been helpful in providing a rationale for [editorial] decisions" [20]. Frances and the *DSM-IV* Task Force maintained a decidedly disengaged stance toward the *DSM-III-R* definition, including it with little revision and crediting it only with helping to guide decisions about marginal cases of disorder—though they give no specific examples of how this was done and Frances' more recent writing casts doubt on whether the *DSM-III-R* definition had any effect at all [26].

Despite the functional irrelevancy of past *DSM* definitions of mental disorder for the construction of the *DSM* itself, early discussion about *DSM-5* revived Spitzer's old hope that a clear definition of mental disorder might play an active role in *DSM-5* decision-making. Rounsaville et al., acknowledging the difficulty and complexity of past attempts at definition, express this hope as follows:

> Despite the difficulties involved, it is desirable that DSM-V should, if at all possible, include a definition of *mental disorder* that can be used as a criterion for assessing potential

candidates for inclusion in the classification, and deletions from it. If for no other reason, this is important because of rising public concern about what is sometimes seen as the progressive medicalization of all problem behaviors and relationships. Even if it proves impossible to formulate a definition of mental disorder that provides an unambiguous criterion for judging all individual candidates, there should at least be no ambiguity about the reason that individual candidate diagnoses are included or excluded [27].

Ten years later, despite some detailed conceptual work on the *DSM-5* definition which was explicitly acknowledged and credited by the DSM-5 Task Force [28], there is no evidence that the *DSM-5* definition has been any more influential in the *DSM-5* revision process than past definitions of mental disorder have been for past editions of the *DSM*. It is notable and ironic, for instance, that Rounsaville et al. grounded the need for a clear definition in "rising public concern about … the progressive medicalization of all problem behaviors and relationships" and that despite this prescient concern, the *DSM-5* revision process has been dogged by a lively and contentious intrapsychiatric debate that *DSM-5* will encourage just this sort of inappropriate medicalization [26]—with no part of this debate influenced by any working definition of "mental disorder." The *DSM-5* Task Force did not act on a public proposal to include a Conceptual Issues Working Group among the other working groups associated with *DSM-5* [29]. As with prior editions of *DSM,* the *DSM-5* definition of "mental disorder" appears to be a late-stage insertion into the manual which, at best, provides some post hoc light on the editorial reasoning of the Task Force. The Task Force could have wrestled deeply with a definition of mental disorder and could have used it as the basis for a substantial revision of the *DSM*—the work of Wakefield, for example, demonstrates how such theory-to-practice critiques might occur [6, 30, 31]—but all indications are that the Task Force did not choose to do so.

If the *DSM* definition of mental disorder has been so marginal in the ongoing revision and articulation of the *DSM,* why should it be included in successive editions of the manual? This is a reasonable question. From a scientific perspective, there seems to be no positive need for a *DSM* definition; if the *DSM* definition were to disappear, very little would change, either in subsequent revisions of *DSM* or in the use of *DSM* by clinicians, researchers, and third-party payers. And it is entirely possible that the definition *will* go away, sooner or later. But for now, in *DSM-5* as in prior editions, the definition remains.

Why does this functionally inconsequential definition of mental disorder remain in the *DSM?* To be sure, no positive reason need exist: the definition may be simply vestigial, carried over from edition to edition because no one has expended the time and energy to remove it. This indeed seems to have been roughly the case for *DSM-IV.* *DSM-5,* though, is more temporally removed from its predecessor than was the case with *DSM-IV,* and the revision process as a whole has been more open to major structural changes and proposals. Though the definition of mental disorder has not by any account been a large part of the Task Force's work, it has been subjected to critical ongoing revision. In this case, it is reasonable to conclude that it serves some function, either ostensive or implicit, within *DSM-5.* I suggest here that the *DSM-5* definition of mental disorder, like its predecessors in *DSM-III, DSM-III-R,* and

DSM-IV, serves a function which is primarily political. To the extent that the definition exerts influence, I argue, it does so by constructing the way that psychiatry is interpreted as a medical specialty—both by psychiatrists themselves and by the larger communities within which psychiatry is practiced—and consequently by constructing the way that individuals in our culture grant authority to psychiatry and psychiatry's diagnostic language.

Seen in historical and political context, the primary function of the *DSM* definition of mental disorder is not to regulate which disorder categories are included in the *DSM* (since it has never explicitly done that), nor to provide an abstract philosophical account of the sort of thing a "mental disorder" is, but rather to delineate the rough boundaries of a clinical "space" within which psychiatry as a medical discipline exercises proper authority and which does not encroach on territory which is socially and politically controversial. There are three specific ways—one by affirmation and two by exclusion—in which the *DSM* definitions (both in *DSM-IV* and in the *DSM-5* definitions proposed to date) attempt to delineate this safe clinical space.

First, the *DSM* definitions use spatial images of depth and interiority to affirm that mental disorders are interior to individuals and that they somehow underlie the distress, disability, and impairment of function which is associated with them. While each of the *DSM* definitions uses slightly different language to convey this, the structural themes are the same: mental disorders reflect dysfunction *in* an individual (or in an individual's cognitions, emotions, and behaviors) which displays itself through subjective distress and/or dysfunction *of* the individual in particular areas of life. *DSM-IV,* for example, specifies that a mental disorder is "a clinically significant behavioral or psychological syndrome or pattern that *occurs in an individual*" and, later, that "whatever its original cause, [a mental disorder] must currently be considered a manifestation of a behavioral, psychological, or biological dysfunction *in* the individual" [italics added]. This distinction between "dysfunction in" an individual and "dysfunction of" the individual in his/her life pursuits, with the "dysfunction in" somehow underlying or causing the "dysfunction of," is important for distinguishing the mental health disciplines (particularly psychiatry) from nonmedical disciplines which also attend to personal distress and social deviance. If psychiatry understood itself simply as a discipline which attended to persons experiencing distress or disability, the *DSM* definition conveys, then psychiatry would have no definitional means by which to distinguish its role from that of other disciplines which also attend to those matters. But fortunately for psychiatry, this is not the case: "mental disorders" turn out not only to be distressing and/or disabling conditions but also conditions which reflect a deeper "dysfunction in" an individual's mental, emotional, and/or cognitive apparatus. Psychiatry is then able to view this deeper "dysfunction in" as the proper object of its expertise. Whether this "dysfunction in" can be demonstrated or located is inconsequential for the *DSM* definition: that it is *presumed* to exist is enough to justify the safe space in which psychiatry can exercise its proper authority.

Second, the *DSM* definitions reinforce the presence of this deeper "dysfunction in" by specifying that a mental disorder must *not* be, as *DSM-IV* puts it, "merely an expectable and culturally sanctioned response to a particular event, for example, the death of a loved one." This negative qualification functions to address the longstanding critical concern that the mental health professions have historically expanded their influence and power by medicalizing aspects of life and behavior which were previously interpreted without the aid of medical models. The *DSM* definitions, by excluding ordinary experience from the concept of mental disorder, attempt to lay this concern to rest.

Third and finally, the *DSM* definitions all make clear that social deviance itself cannot be "mental disorder," and that conflicts between an individual and society are not mental disorders unless the deviance or conflict results—here again—from "dysfunction in the individual." This second negative qualification is necessary to address a second longstanding charge of psychiatry's critics, that psychiatric technology and power function as agents of social control. We may note how much has changed in the *DSM* since its first edition in 1952, in which individuals diagnosed with "sociopathic personality disturbance," of which homosexuality was one example, were understood to be "ill primarily in terms of society and of conformity with the prevailing cultural milieu, and not only in terms of personal discomfort and relations with other individuals" [32]. And it is further worth noting that in certain cultures psychiatric language and authority has indeed been used coercively to suppress social deviants and political dissidents [33]. But the *DSM* definition attempts to ensure readers that none of this is a concern with modern psychiatry: the *DSM* is concerned not with social conflict and deviance but with the underlying dysfunctions of which such conflict and deviance is, at most, a symptom.

In each of these ways, then—through the distinction of "dysfunction in" an individual from "dysfunction of" an individual in his/her life pursuits, through the exclusion of the pathologization of ordinary life, and through the exclusion of the pathologization of social deviance—the *DSM* definitions seek to delineate and map a safe clinical space within which psychiatry can be practiced and in which its authority can be properly exercised. In this mission, they speak differently to the various constituents of the *DSM*. To psychiatrists, they provide a reassuring legitimation of psychiatric authority and a disciplinary reminder of the degree to which psychiatry must continue to conform to modern medical models of diagnosis and treatment (including the modern focus on the individual as the locus of pathology and of treatment). To all mental health professionals, including psychiatrists, they provide a common organizing language which constructs and defines "mental disorder" as a unifying foe, aligning the various mental health disciplines under a common language and a common clinical project. To current or potential patients, they provide reassurance that the diagnostic constructs of the *DSM* are real and that the distress/disability/functional loss which leads them to consider treatment is somehow reflective of a deeper dysfunction "in" themselves, and that seeing a psychiatrist might help to find a fix for this "dysfunction in." To insurers and third-party payers, they reinforce the status of psychiatry as a medical discipline which, naturally, should be treated just as any other medical disciplines are treated. And to would-be critics of psychiatry, they provide at least ostensive defense against the most common anti-psychiatric critiques.

There is No Safe Space for Psychiatry: Why the *DSM* Definitions Fail

So far in this chapter I have argued that the *DSM* definition of mental disorder evolved in a particular sociohistorical context in which psychiatry was seeking to burnish its credibility as a medical discipline against internal and external critics who were challenging psychiatry's authority and legitimacy. I have argued that Spitzer initially proposed a forerunner of the *DSM-III* definition as a direct result of his involvement in the controversy surrounding the diagnostic status of homosexuality, and with the hope that a clear definition of mental disorder could guide nosological decisions during the *DSM-III* revision process. I have argued that despite Spitzer's hope, no *DSM* definition of mental disorder, including that in *DSM-III*, has ever served the regulative role that Spitzer envisioned; at best, the *DSM* definitions have provided a rough post hoc account of the general nosological commitments of the *DSM* architects. They have not been and are not, by any account, essential to the construction and revision of the various *DSM* editions. They do, however, serve a distinct *political* function: to conceptually delineate a safe clinical space within which psychiatry can exercise its authority.

If the *DSM* definitions were conceptually and logically successful in delineating this safe clinical space for psychiatry, this would be an incalculable gift to psychiatry and to all of the mental health disciplines. If "mental disorder" could be clearly and logically defined, and the proper boundaries of psychiatry's authority successfully demarcated, the long and complex struggle of psychiatry to legitimate itself within the pantheon of medical disciplines and to establish its legitimacy with the broader public would be effectively over. Psychiatry could pursue its proper work—investigating, preventing, treating, and ultimately eliminating "mental disorders"—with boldness and authority. The problem for the *DSM* and for its communities of reception, however, is that the *DSM* definitions of mental disorder do not successfully establish any such safe clinical space. Far from defending psychiatry against anti-psychiatric critique, the *DSM* definitions in fact display the high degree to which psychiatric diagnosis is both value-laden and politically contestable. There are at least three reasons why this is the case.

The first reason that the *DSM* definitions fail to delineate a safe clinical space for psychiatry is that the central distinction which they make—the distinction between the distress/disability/functional loss *of* the individual and dysfunction *in* the individual which causes the "dysfunction of"—is at present indemonstrable with regard to most of the *DSM* mental disorder constructs. The problem is not, of course, a matter of recognizing the subjective distress, disability, or loss of function which brings patients into psychiatric care. That is clearly and self-evidently demonstrable. The problem, rather, is in meaningfully identifying and describing specific "dysfunction in the individual" which correlates to or causes this "dysfunction of." In certain specific psychopathological cases—in Alzheimer's-type dementia, for example (or, in the likely *DSM-5* nomenclature, "Major Neurocognitive Disorder Due to Alzheimer's Disease")—this distinction is clearly meaningful even if the specific neuroanatomical lesions which correlate with the clinical phenotype of cognitive disorder are not (yet) able to be seen in vivo. In the case of Alzheimer's disease, well-defined, highly correlated neural lesions (whatever their cause) are associated with "dysfunction in" the brain which correlates closely with the "dysfunction of" the person in his/her life projects. But in the case of most current *DSM* mental disorders, there is simply no reliable and noncircular way to identify "dysfunction in" without recourse to the "dysfunction of" which brings a patient into treatment. Sometimes this is because no biomarkers or psychological endophenotypes have been identified for specific disorders. Sometimes this is because particular biomarkers or psychological phenotypes have been correlated with particular disorders, but the way that these markers function is so poorly understood that a judgment of "dysfunction" would be premature and unintelligible, lacking an account of "proper function." Sometimes this is because the teleological frames used to make judgments about dysfunction (such as the evolutionary theory of Wakefield) are themselves speculative and contestable [34].

All of these are, of course, surmountable obstacles—it is conceptually possible (though doubtful, for reasons given below) that a future science of psychiatry will have developed robust bottom-up accounts of biological and psychological function which are sufficient for the identification and recognition of "dysfunction in the individual." But that is simply not how things work right now in the clinical practice of psychiatry. In the modern practice of psychiatry, in most cases, clinicians recognize the presence of distress or "dysfunction of" an individual, *infer* the presence of a "dysfunction in" from this "dysfunction of," and then establish a treatment plan targeted at the amelioration of the distress and/or "dysfunction of" the patient. It is generally not possible to clearly describe a "dysfunction in" which can be distinguished from this "dysfunction of."

In itself, this inability to distinguish "dysfunction of" an individual from an underlying "dysfunction in" an individual is not particularly important: psychiatrists can care well for patients, and patients can flourish, without any need for such a distinction. But if "dysfunction in" cannot in practice be identified apart from "dysfunction of," the *DSM* definitions of mental disorder are rendered powerless to guard psychiatric nosology against the medicalization of ordinary life and of social deviance. The definitions are in fact shown to be absurdly circular. How is it, a critic might ask, that Disorder A is properly a mental disorder and not simply a conflict between an individual and society? The definitions respond: because the conflict results from a "dysfunction in" the individual. But how, the critic might respond, do we know that such a "dysfunction in" exists? The definitions respond: because its presence is inferred from the distress, disability, and "dysfunction of" the person in his/her life context. And so the efforts of the *DSM* definitions to guard psychiatric nosology against the medicalization of ordinary life and social deviance are seen, in many cases, to be circular and therefore vacuous.

The second reason that the *DSM* definitions fail to delineate a safe clinical space for psychiatry is that "function" is and likely will always be a socially contestable concept. Writing about the homosexuality debate of the 1970s, for example, Robert Spitzer recognized clearly that even his proposed definition for *DSM-III* would not resolve fundamental debates regarding the diagnostic status of homosexuality: it would only help to clarify them. The question of whether homosexuality represented an "impairment in one or more important areas of functioning," Spitzer wrote, begged the question of what the norm of "function" is taken to be. If *sexual* functioning is the norm, without regard to same-sex or opposite-sex preference, then homosexuality per se is no functional impairment. But if *heterosexual* functioning is taken as the norm—as it was, for instance, in the disease model of Kendell [16]—then homosexuality is indeed a dysfunction, and therefore a disorder. Although modern psychiatry no longer debates the diagnostic status of homosexuality, Spitzer's point holds true for all disorder-judgments which make any recourse to normative function: "function" is a teleological (or at least contextual) concept which, when used normatively, calls for an account of how circumstances *should be* or *would be* if a thing were "functioning" correctly [35–38]. Assigning a judgment of "dysfunction," that is, entails some conception of what proper function looks like. This, then, begs the question of authority: who decides what counts as proper function, and how are disagreements about proper function to be arbitrated? Here again, the *DSM* definitions of mental disorder do not rescue psychiatric diagnosis from sociopolitical critique and controversy: rather, in invoking the concept of function, they display the degree to which psychiatric diagnosis depends on normative standards which are themselves socially contestable [39].

Third and finally, the *DSM* definitions fail psychiatry through their consistent stipulation that mental disorders occur "in an individual" rather than in any larger social context. This insistence on methodological individualism is nowhere defended in the definitions nor in the text of the *DSM* itself; it is simply stipulated. This stipulation of individualism is not so much a logical failure as it is an imaginative failure, constraining the ways that psychiatry understands the role of the individual with respect to his/her social environment, and the ways in which mental disorders are framed and conceptualized [40]. Politically, individualism is convenient for psychiatry: it preserves and justifies the dominant dyadic models of treatment, structurally aligns psychiatric diagnoses with other medical diagnoses, and helps to reinforce the claim that psychiatry does not pathologize conflicts between an individual and society unless this conflict results from a "dysfunction in the individual." But in embracing methodological individualism, the *DSM* binds itself to western (and particularly American) models of the self [41] which, in turn, both hinder imaginative conceptual work about the nature of mental disorders and, importantly, leave the *DSM* vulnerable to charges that its diagnostic constructs are themselves culture-bound [42].

How to Go On Without a Definition of Mental Disorder: Toward a Psychiatry Without Foundations

The four-decade-old quest within American psychiatry to formulate a clear definition of "mental disorder" for use in the *DSM*, birthed in the social and political milieu of the 1970s and continued through successive editions of the *DSM*, has in many ways been a fruitful and useful process. It has rendered psychiatrists more articulate about the thorny conceptual questions which permeate psychiatric research and practice. It has engendered a great deal of thoughtful debate within the psychiatric, philosophical, and psychological literature. But it has not produced—and likely will not produce in the foreseeable future—a definition of mental disorder that successfully demarcates a safe clinical space for psychiatric diagnosis and treatment which is both regulative for nosological decisions and capable of safeguarding psychiatry against social and political critique. Far from fulfilling these tasks, the *DSM* definitions of mental disorder are at best irrelevant and at worst circular, misleading, and constraining. And so, I suggest, they should be retired. Future editions of the *DSM,* at least until the development of much more detailed and robust ground-up accounts of neurobiological and psychological function than we have now, should not include a definition of mental disorder. And if and when any future definition makes recourse to the concepts of "function" or "dysfunction," the manual should make explicitly clear how proper "function" is understood and framed, *who decides* what "proper function" is, and how disputes about the meaning of "proper function" will be arbitrated.

Given the political weight of the present definition within the *DSM,* revocation of the definition of "mental disorder" from future editions of the *DSM* is not a politically appealing prospect. It would surely be seen by some critics of psychiatry as a concession of defeat. It would render the *DSM* more vulnerable to charges that its classification is arbitrary and nonsystematic, and that the *DSM* reflects social judgments about the use of psychiatry more than it reflects any foundational theory of psychiatry's proper role with regard to human suffering. The *DSM* would appear to be an artifact of *bricolage,* a catalogue of conditions in which psychiatry happens to take some interest and which have historically been constructed as proper domains of psychiatry's authority. And it would remove any systematic, a priori way to defend psychiatry against the common charges that psychiatry medicalizes ordinary life and that psychiatry medicalizes social deviance. At the very least, removal of the *DSM* definition would encourage critical thought and analysis as to how this sort of medicalization might occur.

All of this is true—and it would be healthy, both for psychiatric diagnostic classification and for psychiatry as a whole. As I have argued in this chapter, the *DSM* definition of mental disorder neither successfully defines mental disorder nor provides a safe clinical space for psychiatry to exercise its authority. It only *seems* to do so, and therefore serves as a conceptual analgesic which, far from resolving conceptual problems related to psychiatry's proper role, only renders hard and difficult questions less likely to be addressed. But psychiatry can, and should, go on without such a definition. Without the cover of a definition of mental disorder, contemporary psychiatry would neither be discredited nor rendered incoherent. It would simply be seen for what it is: a scientifically, morally, and philosophically complex practice in which practitioners, trained in particular ways of understanding human beings and in the use of particular forms of technique, do the best that they can to attend helpfully to persons whose particular configurations of behavior, cognition, emotion, and experience are judged, by a process of social construction and narration, to warrant their care and attention. It would be seen as a lively and diverse discipline with no foundational, unifying theory, despite many hard-fought attempts to develop one. Precisely *because* of its scientific, moral, and philosophical complexity, it would be seen as ever-vulnerable to self-aggrandizement and to manipulation by forces external to it, with the consequent need to remain vigilant, self-critical, and responsive to feedback from its various constituents. A psychiatry willing to go on without a definition of mental disorder would be a psychiatry without foundations—but since the present foundations cannot hold the weight placed upon them, that is just where psychiatry needs to be.

References

1. Stagnitti M. Antidepressants prescribed by medical doctors in office based and outpatient settings by specialty for the U.S. civilian noninstitutionalized population, 2002 and 2005. Agency for Healthcare Research and Quality, Medical Expenditure Panel Survey, Statistical Brief #206.
2. Insel T, Quirion R. Psychiatry as a clinical neuroscience discipline. JAMA. 2005;294: 2221–4.
3. American Psychiatric Association. What is psychiatry? [Internet]. 2012 [cited 2012 Sept 9]. http://www.psychiatry.org/about-apa--psychiatry/more-about-psychiatry.
4. Bayer R. Homosexuality and American psychiatry: the politics of diagnosis. Princeton, NJ: Princeton University Press; 1981.
5. Elliott C. Better than well: American medicine meets the American dream. New York: W. W. Norton; 2003.
6. Horwitz AV, Wakefield JC. The loss of sadness: how psychiatry transformed normal sorrow into depressive disorder. New York: Oxford University Press; 2007.
7. Gert B, Culver CM. Sex, immorality, and mental disorders. J Med Philos. 2009;34:487–95.
8. Szasz T. The myth of mental illness: foundations of a theory of personal conduct. Revised ed. New York: Harper & Row; 1974.
9. Foucault M. History of madness. London: Routledge; 2006 [J. Murphy, trans].
10. Mayes R, Horwitz AV. DSM-III and the revolution in the classification of mental illness. J Hist Behav Sci. 2005;41:249–67.
11. Goffman E. Asylums: essays on the social situations of mental patients and other inmates. Piscataway, NJ: Aldine Transaction; 2007.
12. Kesey K. One flew over the cuckoo's nest. New York: Penguin Classics; 2002.
13. Rosenhan DL. On being sane in insane places. Science. 1973;179:250–8.
14. American Psychiatric Association. Diagnostic and statistical manual of mental disorders. 3rd ed. Washington, DC: American Psychiatric Association; 1980.
15. Scadding JG. Diagnosis: the clinician and the computer, Lancet. 1967;7521:877–82.
16. Kendell RE. The concept of disease and its implications for psychiatry. Br J Psychiatry. 1975;127:305–15.
17. Klein DF. A proposed definition of mental illness. In: Spitzer RL, Klein DF, editors. Critical issues in psychiatric diagnosis. New York: Raven; 1978.
18. Spitzer RL. The diagnostic status of homosexuality in DSM-III: a reformulation of the issues. Am J Psychiatry. 1981;138:210–5.
19. Spitzer RL, Endicott J. Medical and mental disorder: proposed definition and criteria. In: Spitzer RL, Klein DF, editors. Critical issues in psychiatric diagnosis. New York: Raven; 1978.
20. Spitzer RL, Williams JBW. The definition and diagnosis of mental disorder. In: Gove WR, editor. Deviance and mental illness. Beverly Hills: Sage; 1982.

21. Spitzer RL, Williams JBW, Skodol AE. DSM-III: the major achievements and an overview. Am J Psychiatry. 1980;137:151–64.
22. American Psychiatric Association. Diagnostic and statistical manual of mental disorders. 3rd revised ed. Washington, DC: American Psychiatric Association; 1987.
23. American Psychiatric Association. Diagnostic and statistical manual of mental disorders. 4th ed. Washington, DC: American Psychiatric Association; 1994.
24. Frances A, Pincus HA, Widiger TA, Davis WW, First MB. DSM-IV: work in progress. Am J Psychiatry. 1990;147:1439–48.
25. Definition of a mental disorder [Internet]. 2012 [cited 2 Oct 2012]. http://www.dsm5.org/proposedrevision/Pages/proposedrevision.aspx?rid=465.
26. Phillips J, Frances A, Cerullo MA, Chardavoyne J, Decker HS, First MB, et al. The six most essential questions in psychiatric diagnosis: a pluralogue Part 1: conceptual and definitional issues in psychiatric diagnosis. Philosophy, Ethics, and Humanities in Medicine. 2012;7:2. doi:10.1186/1747-5341-7-3.
27. Rounsaville BJ, Alarcon RD, Andrews G, Jackson JS, Kendell RE, Kendler K. Basic nomenclature issues for DSM-V. In: Kupfer DA, First MB, Regier DA, editors. A research agenda for DSM-V. Washington, DC: American Psychiatric Association; 2002.
28. Stein DJ, Phillips KA, Bolton D, Fulford KWM, Sadler JZ, Kendler KS. What is a mental/psychiatric disorder? From DSM-IV to DSM-V. Psychol Med. 2010;40:759–65.
29. Kendler KS, Appelbaum PS, Bell CC, Fulford KWM, Ghaemi SN, Shaffner KF, et al. Issues for DSM-V: DSM-V should include a conceptual issues workgroup. Am J Psychiatry. 2008;165:174–5.
30. Wakefield JC. The concept of mental disorder: on the boundary between biological facts and social values. Am Psychol. 1992;47:373–88.
31. Wakefield JC. Diagnosing DSM-IV—Part I: DSM-IV and the concept of disorder. Behav Res Ther. 1997;35:633–49.
32. American Psychiatric Association. Diagnostic and statistical manual: mental disorders. Washington, DC: American Psychiatric Association Mental Hospital Service; 1952.
33. Fulford KWM, Smirnov AYU, Snow E. Concepts of disease and the abuse of psychiatry in the USSR. Br J Psychiatry. 1993;162:801–10.
34. Bolton D. What is mental disorder? An essay in philosophy, science, and values. Oxford: Oxford University Press; 2008.
35. Sadler JZ, Agich GJ. Diseases, functions, values, and psychiatric classification. PPP. 1995;2:219–31.
36. Wakefield JC. Dysfunction as a value-free concept: a reply to Sadler and Agich. PPP. 1995;2:233–46.
37. Fulford KWM. Nine variations and a coda on the theme of an evolutionary definition of dysfunction. J Abnorm Psychol. 1999;108:412–20.
38. Fulford KWM. Teleology without tears: naturalism, neo-naturalism, and evaluationism in the analysis of function statements in biology (and a bet on the twenty-first century). PPP. 2000;7:77–94.
39. Sadler JZ. Values and psychiatric diagnosis. New York: Oxford University Press; 2005.
40. Blazer DG. The age of melancholy: 'major depression' and its social origins. New York: Routledge; 2005.
41. Kirmayer LJ. Psychotherapy and the cultural concept of the person. Transcult Psychiatry. 2007;44:232–57.
42. Chen Y, Nettles ME, Chen S. Rethinking dependent personality disorder: comparing different human relatedness in cultural contexts. J Nerv Ment Dis. 2009;197:793–800.

Chapter 5
Establishing Normative Validity for Scientific Psychiatric Nosology: The Significance of Integrating Patient Perspectives

Douglas Porter

Introduction

The potential for patients to contribute to a scientific psychiatric nosology is further reaching than is commonly recognized. It extends all the way into the heart of the science of nosology, into the establishment of scientific validity. This assertion may appear strange in view of the fact that the neo-Kraepelinian notion of validity, so influential in contemporary psychiatric nosology, was felt to place the issue of validity, at last, on a firm empirical scientific footing. But it would be a mistake to equate an empirical footing with a transcendence of normative questions about the right way to proceed. It is not a matter of nosology either being empirical or normative. Instead nosology entails a mixture of the descriptive and the prescriptive. When carefully examined, it becomes apparent that neo-Kraepelinian notions of validity are underdetermined by empirical truth claims and must be supplemented by normative claims about what nosology ought to accomplish. When the normative assumptions that guide neo-Kraepelinian nosology are made explicit it becomes equally apparent that there are alternative ways of conceptualizing nosology that are commensurate with the empirical data. Normative elements are not an extra-scientific appendage of nosology. There is simply a normative dimension to the science of nosology. The normative dimension of science often makes scientists uncomfortable because it entails evaluative elements. Positivist equations of the evaluative with the subjective and the arbitrary are still very influential in scientific circles, and scientists are used to justifying empirical truth claims about the world, not normative truth claims about the right way to proceed. The philosophical work of Jurgen Habermas is a helpful antidote here because, counter to a stance of value skepticism or relativism, Habermas maintains that normative judgments about the

D. Porter (✉)
Central City Behavioral Health Center, 2221 Phillip Street, 70113 New Orleans, LA, USA
e-mail: douglasporter@cox.net

J. Paris and J. Phillips (eds.), *Making the DSM-5: Concepts and Controversies*,
DOI 10.1007/978-1-4614-6504-1_5, © Springer Science+Business Media New York 2013

right way to proceed are susceptible to falsifiable validity claims. Habermas establishes a procedural notion of normative validity that would safeguard the normative issues in nosology from being resolved in an arbitrary or coercive manner. This procedural notion of normative validity points toward the depth of importance of patient participation for the science of nosology. The fact that normative issues form an essential part of nosology means that we should remain skeptical toward any claims for the validity of the science that ignore the normative dimension of the science while attending solely to empirical issues.

Channels for public input were made available during the development of the Diagnostic and Statistical Manual of Mental Disorders 5 (DSM-5). Input came from patients, family members of patients, patient advocacy groups as well as other stakeholders. Leadership of the DSM-5 revision process cited numerous positives that resulted from patient contributions including prevention of the use of pejorative terms and the prevention of unintended consequences such as increasing stigma and interfering with access to care [1]. The level of patient contribution to the DSM-5 can be seen as the culmination of a growing trend in the most recent formulations of the DSM toward greater democratization and transparency in the process of development. But the development of the DSM-5 was also guided by a self-conscious drive toward developing diagnoses with greater validity [2]. The DSM-5 leadership adopted a largely neo-Kraepelinian conception of validity that has been a guiding force for psychiatric nosology since the development of DSM-III [3]. This conception of validity is contestable and, as it currently stands, actually acts to conceal the depth of potential benefit from patient participation in the development of psychiatric nosology. In order to understand this we must retrace the logic of neo-Kraepelinian and to some extinct Kraepelinian conceptions of valid diagnostic constructs.

The Atheoretical Theory of the Neo-Kraepelinians

The term "neo-Kraepelinian" refers to a school of thought emanating from a group of psychiatrists at Washington University in the late 1960s and early 1970s. The namesake of this school was Emil Kraepelin, a preeminent psychiatrist whose theories were immensely influential at the beginning of the twentieth century. The neo-Kraepelinian school of thought was critical of the psychoanalytic influence on psychiatry and wanted to move psychiatry toward a medical model with a greater emphasis on biology [4]. An important aspect of the neo-Kraepelinian turn was a return to an emphasis on clinical description. Kraepelin was renowned for his careful empirical work in the description of the signs and symptoms of mental illness. Organizing nosology on the basis of a description of signs and symptoms without specific reference to etiology in DSM-III could be seen as a neo-Kraepelinian turn in psychiatric nosology. It certainly marked a significant conceptual shift from the organizing principles of DSM-II where psychoanalytically oriented conceptions of etiology were contained within the definitions of mental disorders [5]. The neo-Kraepelinian conception of validity was spearheaded by Robins and Guze prior to the publication of DSM-III. Their seminal paper on diagnostic validity published in 1970 [6] pioneered the use of external validators as a means of establishing the validity of a diagnostic construct. Specifically Robins and Guze stated that a diagnostic construct should be validated by family studies, course of illness, clinical description, laboratory studies, and differential diagnosis. External validators afford evidence that diagnostic constructs provide relevant information not already contained in the definition of the diagnostic construct. As such they could be interpreted as providing evidence of the pragmatic value of the diagnostic construct. But, there is good reason to question the adoption of a "validity through pragmatic value" stance on the part of the neo-Kraepelinians. It was perhaps the move away from psychoanalytic theory that motivated Robins and Guze [6] to announce that their concept of validity was not based upon "a priori principles." But it would be more accurate to state that their notion of validity is based upon different a priori principles than those of psychoanalysis and, it should be noted, different a priori principles than those of pragmatism.

There is a productive tradition within medicine of moving from the description of a characteristic pattern of signs and symptoms in the form of a syndrome to the eventual discovery of the etiology of the syndrome. When the etiology is discovered the syndrome attains the status of a disease entity. The term "disease" is, of course, also used within medicine to refer to illnesses where there is no knowledge of etiology. But there is reason to believe that this historical notion of the syndrome as a stepping stone on the way to disease is theoretically operational in the thinking of the neo-Kraepelinians and compatible with the thinking of Kraepelin himself. Kraepelin, in his 1899 textbook, asserted his belief that "cases arising from the same causes would always have to present the same symptoms and the same post-mortem result" [7]. If this holds true then the characteristic patterns of signs and symptoms described by a syndrome could be seen as mapping onto or representing characteristic biological changes which in turn represent genetic sources of etiology. In this light, the external validators developed by Robins and Guze take on a different form of significance than evidence of pragmatic value. They can be seen as evidence that the syndrome described is "valid" in the sense that it represents a characteristic biological change in the brain with a genetic etiology at root. As noted earlier, Robins and Guze elaborated five external validators: family studies of heredity, clinical description, clinical course, differential diagnosis, and lab studies. Robins and Guze made it clear that a diagnostic construct could only be considered "fully validated" [6] if all five validators apply. If a construct represented a disease in the Kraepelinian sense of a biologically determined syndrome with an underlying genetic etiology then we would indeed expect all five validators to line up on that particular construct.

Neo-Kraepelinians Compton and Guze were quite explicit that the notion of validity first elaborated by Robins and Guze was part and parcel of a "medical model" of psychiatry that could be differentiated from a biopsychosocial model, for example, because, "the brain and how brain mechanisms are related to functional impairment would be considered the first goal of medical-model psychiatry" [8]. Yet they continued to regard themselves as working on the basis of observation

alone without any theoretical assumptions, leading to the seemingly self contradictory statement, "The medical model is without a priori theory, but does consider
brain mechanisms to be a priority" [8]. It could be that the belief that mental syndromes map seamlessly onto specific biological abnormalities is not regarded by
neo-Kraepelinians as a theoretical assumption that can be called into question
because it is held as a matter of faith that this is the nature of "reality." Theoretical
assumptions cannot be called into question if they entail an unreflective commitment to an implicit ontology. This seems to have been confirmed by Kendell and
Jablensky [9] when they referred to Kraepelin as a "disease realist," where a *real*
disease is one in which we understand the causal mechanisms behind the signs and
symptoms and validity can be considered synonymous with "delineating a specific, necessary, and sufficient biological mechanism" [9]. Kendell and Jablensky
readily acknowledged the implicit "disease entity" assumption at play in the work
of Robins and Guze. It should be noted that Robert Spitzer, the chief architect of
DSM-III, protested against accusations that the DSM favored a biological perspective. He held that the descriptive approach of the DSM facilitated etiological pluralism. He further stated external validators were evidence of the usefulness of a
diagnostic construct (as opposed to evidence that it represented an underlying biological entity or mechanism). He specifically used the term "clinical utility (validity)" [5], implying that validity and clinical utility are synonymous. Kendell and
Jablensky were highly critical of Spitzer's pragmatic definition of validity stating
that valid diagnoses must be clearly differentiated from diagnoses that merely
have utility. For Kendell and Jablensky syndromes may be considered valid only
insofar as there is evidence that "natural boundaries" [9] exist between them. In
stark contrast to Spitzer's identification of validity and pragmatic utility, Kendell
and Jablensky identify the pragmatic with the arbitrary, asserting that in the
absence of natural boundaries, boundaries must "be decided arbitrarily on pragmatic grounds" [9].

The diagnostic constructs contained heretofore in the DSM have not been validated in the sense delineated by Robins and Guze, a fact readily recognized by the
DSM-5 leadership [3]. But, this fact has not been interpreted by the DSM-5 leadership as reason to call the neo-Kraepelinian concept of validity into question. Instead
there appears to be ample evidence that neo-Kraepelinian theoretical commitments
remain largely intact. We could imagine ourselves to be reading one of Kraepelin's
texts when Regier declares that the DSM-5 objective of facilitating "research
exploring the etiology and pathophysiology of mental disorders" is tantamount to "a
renewed focus on the validity of diagnoses" [2]. When *diverse* (emphasis mine) top-
ics in depression research are noted to include "preclinical animal models, genetics,
pathophysiology, functional imaging, clinical treatment, epidemiology, prevention,
medical comorbidity, and public health implications" [2], I think it is fair to conclude that the medical model extolled by Compton and Guze has remained very
much at work in the development of DSM-5. The psychosocial aspects of illness are
largely marginalized and diversity within the biological sciences appears to be all
the diversity that is needed.

The Pragmatic Turn

Neo-Kraepelinian thinking may equate the pragmatic with the arbitrary but it is possible to invert this logic and call into question the pragmatic value of maintaining neo-Kraepelinian theoretical assumptions. Karl Jaspers [10] wrote in 1913 with skepticism about Kraepelin's assumption that psychological forms would map seamlessly onto cerebral pathology which would map seamlessly onto specific genetic etiologies. This skepticism was founded not only on the historical failure to discern specific etiologies for specific patterns of psychopathology, but also on the realization that in the case of syphilis, where the specific etiology of psychopathology is known, a great diversity of symptomatic presentations results. Jaspers proposed "ideal types" [10] as an alternative means of categorizing mental disorder. As opposed to conceiving of a syndrome as representing a concrete thing or essential process, ideal types are seen to abstract a few salient features from the myriad of empirical data available on the basis of pragmatic interests. The use of ideal types in nosology has contemporary advocates [11, 12], and Peter Zachar [13] has delineated a practical kind model for classification that has much in common with the notion of ideal types. This model emphasizes that those decisions about where to draw the conceptual lines in nosology will change depending upon our pragmatic interests. It is important to note that the discovery of a singular determining etiology for a mental disorder would likely have tremendous pragmatic value, not only prognostically but quite possibly leading to the development of therapeutic interventions. As such, "real diseases" in the traditional sense advocated by neo-Kraepelinians may certainly be accommodated by a practical kind model. Jaspers [10], for example, noted that even in the absence of "real diseases" working scientifically as if there were mental diseases could yield pragmatically useful information. But Jaspers found the disease model neither necessary nor sufficient and therefore advocated a plurality of approaches to study the complex subject of psychopathology. Because a practical kinds model does not have a theoretical/ontological commitment to the traditional disease concept it can entertain different manners of conceptualizing disorder and call into question the pragmatic value of insisting upon a disease model if and when that seems to lead us further and further afield from matters with clinical relevance. A pragmatic approach transcends the mindset that illness is either entirely a biological matter or not biological at all. As such it can incorporate relevant contributions not only from the biological and social sciences but from philosophy and the humanities as well [14].

The scientific work of Kenneth Kendler has emphasized that in addition to biological factors, psychological, social, and cultural factors can be seen to have an impact on the development of psychopathology. These factors do not work in isolation or in a simple linear, additive manner. Instead they influence each other in a complex manner that belies a simplistic singularly determining etiology story for mental disorder. For example a genetic disposition to alcoholism may be modified by the cultural acceptability of alcohol use, policies of taxation, or simply by witnessing the horrible toll that alcoholism exacted on one's parents [15]. Clinically, are we going to conclude that alcoholism is not a "real" medical problem because biological approaches only tell part of the story? The mindset that holds that mental disorders are all biological or not biological at all simply does not put us in the best position to understand the complex phenomena that fall under the rubric of mental disorder. Kendler [16] underscores that alcoholism is not an exception in this regard. In general, psychiatric disorders lend themselves to explanatory pluralism. This pluralism stands as a stark alternative to seeing nosology as the neo-Kraepelinians did. At the time of the advent of DSM-III there seemed to be essentially a choice between psychoanalytic mechanistic forms of explanation or biological mechanistic forms of explanation [5]. The picture that emerges from Kendler's work is that biological approaches to understanding mental disorder have limited explanatory power and we are in a better position to understand mental disorders if we take a pluralistic approach.

Schaffner [17] noted that genetic determination of behavior appears to be an oversimplification even in the simplest behaviors exemplified by the simplest forms of organisms. In Schaffner's studies of nematode behavior, genetic behavioral dispositions unfolded differently in different environmental contexts. As such it should not come as a surprise that the diagnostic construct for schizophrenia that is best validated by course of illness is a narrower construct than that best validated by family history [18]. A broader definition of schizophrenia includes what the narrow definition would exclude and define as different disorders, schizotypal personality, and the affective psychoses for example. The broader definition is better able to accommodate a genetic disposition that can unfold in a different manner depending upon environmental contingencies. The narrow definition has more specific prognostic ramifications. The fact that different validators point toward different constructs makes neither the narrow diagnostic construct nor the broad diagnostic construct valid by the standards of Robins and Guze. It is important to note the different potential theoretical responses to empirical evidence of the lack of neo-Kraepelinian validity in the current DSM nosology. One can reject entirely the value of syndromal medicine for nosology and instead pursue a neuro-circuitry first and foremost strategy. This appears to be the guiding supposition of the Research Domain Criteria (RDoC) project being funded by the National Institute of Mental Health [19]. One can attempt to reform syndromal nosology in a more dimensional direction in order to better reflect the underlying biological etiology. This appears to be the strategy of the DSM-5 leadership [3]. Thinkers with a pragmatic orientation can assert that no one diagnostic construct can be all things to all people, and accordingly conclude that the hegemony of any singular system of nosology is unjustified. Instead they call for a more pluralistic approach to nosology [20]. Indeed, it is possible to endorse both the RDoC and the DSM approaches as pragmatically "valid," the DSM approach having greater clinical utility but the RDoC having potential value for scientific research regarding etiology.

The Normative Turn

The potential for multiple theoretical responses to what is recognized as the same empirical fact underscores the evaluative dimension of the science of nosology. Kenneth Kendler [18] emphasized the normative issues involved in the science of nosology that are not simply resolved by the collection of data. Which theoretical assumptions should we adopt, which explanations should take priority, which validators have more practical importance? The notion of a *valid* diagnostic construct entails multiple evaluative judgments of salience. Evaluative issues were always present in neo-Kraepelinian nosology but they remained implicit. With the pragmatic turn evaluative issues become explicit and therefore visibly contestable. Because the pragmatic turn clarifies the evaluative dimensions of the science of nosology it puts us in position to examine the ethical dimensions of the science of nosology. Are the normative judgments that are being rendered ethically justifiable? The philosophical work of Jurgen Habermas on discourse ethics is helpful here because in addition to recognizing falsifiable validity claims about empirical aspects of the world, Habermas holds that the resolution of normative issues are also subject to falsifiable validity claims. Habermas's theoretical work is diverse and complex and an extensive examination of his ideas is well beyond the scope of this chapter. Nonetheless a brief excursion into Habermas's ideas is justified because he clarifies a position that stands in opposition to the belief that the resolution of value judgments is hopelessly subjective, arbitrary, and irrational. Habermas's philosophical ideas remain relatively unfamiliar to American thinkers, but they stand in a neo-Kantian tradition that is compatible with the traditional precepts of medical ethics. In addition, Habermas establishes normative validity through a process that is analogous in many ways to the process the influential philosopher of science Helen Longino devised to justify scientific claims to objectivity. As such the ideas employed by Habermas in his theory of normative validity should be relatively accessible to a broad audience.

Habermas is "neo-Kantian" in the sense that he adopts the Kantian premise that moral values should be differentiated from other ethical values on the basis of their universal significance [21]. While there may be a plurality of ethical views of "the good life," there is a universal moral imperative to respect a person's capacity to reason and develop a notion of the good life [22]. Kant formalized the moral imperative to universally respect free and equal moral persons with his categorical imperative to treat all people as ends in themselves and never merely as a means to fulfill another person's needs [23]. Habermas adopts Kant's moral imperative for universal respect for persons and notes accordingly that institutional norms should be acceptable to all the people affected by those institutions. Habermas states that "valid norms must deserve recognition by all concerned" [24] and formalizes this in a principle of universalization. For every valid norm: "All affected can accept the consequences and the side effects its general observance can be expected to have for the satisfaction of everyone's interests" [24].

But, Habermas is critical of Kant's and much later John Rawls's [25] attempts to monologically justify the universalizability of a norm on the basis of a thought experiment. It simply places too much burden on one thinker to determine that a norm is acceptable to all affected parties. Instead Habermas invokes the importance of an inclusive deliberative democratic process as a means of establishing/confirming this acceptability. Habermas posits a discourse principle where: "Only those norms can claim to be valid that meet (or could meet) with the approval of all affected in their capacity as participants in a practical discourse" [24].

Habermas is, of course, aware that empirical cases of consensus may very well be invalid if, for example, they are secured through coercive acts of manipulation. Habermas introduces rules of argumentation in order to minimize coercion in discourse:

> Every subject with the competence to speak and act is allowed to take part in a discourse.
> Everyone is allowed to question any assertion whatever.
> Everyone is allowed to introduce any assertion whatever into the discourse.
> Everyone is allowed to express his attitudes, desires, and needs [24].

Helen Longino [26] has noted the strong parallels in Habermas's procedural approach to securing normative validity with her own procedural approach to securing objective knowledge in the sciences. For Longino objectivity in science hinges upon four criteria:

> There must be recognized avenues for the criticism of evidence, of methods, and of assumptions and reasoning;
> There must exist shared standards that critics can invoke;
> The community as a whole must be responsive to such criticism;
> Intellectual authority must be shared equally among qualified practitioners [26].

The reason for the similarity in approach is that both thinkers are trying to minimize coercive practices so that the persuasive force of the better argument is the only force at play. This holds true whether the discourse involves empirical assertions or normative assertions.

To some extent Kant's categorical imperative to treat people as ends in themselves has already been institutionalized in the practice of medicine. The categorical imperative grounds the moral significance of the principle of autonomy guiding the practice of informed consent in medicine [27]. Much ado is often made in medical ethics of the conflicting demands of principles of autonomy which underscore the importance of treating a person as self-determined and principles of beneficence that demand physicians act in the best interests of their patients. But, the truth is respect for autonomy typically furthers the interest in beneficence. The moral significance of beneficence is underscored by the vulnerability created by illness and the imbalance of power seen in the clinical encounter. The principle of autonomy clarifies that in order to act in the best interests of a patient medical knowledge must be applied in a manner that accords with the patient's conception of their best interests [28]. The practice of informed consent is a further means of ensuring that the vulnerability and imbalance of power created by illness does not prevent beneficent medical practice. If medical knowledge were a value-neutral matter then the normative issues involved would be exhausted by the consensual application of that knowledge in the clinical encounter. But, as we have seen from our exploration of the theoretical issues at stake in nosology, the development of medical knowledge is far from value-neutral. Edmund Pellegrino and David Thomasma [29] have noted that medicine is a profession insofar as physicians profess knowledge of *value* to their patients. "Practical" interests are in the eye of the beholder. Medical knowledge has the potential to be developed according to practical interests, for example guild or industrial interests, which diverge from patient interests. If medical knowledge were developed according to guild interests as opposed to patient interests, the knowledge could be empirically valid and of practical value, yet the knowledge would be unjust and therefore normatively invalid. This underscores the fact that practice of informed consent at the bedside may be necessary but it is not sufficient to ensure patient autonomy. The consensual application of unjust knowledge hardly secures patient autonomy.

Transcribing the notion of autonomy to the institutional level entails developing institutional norms that accommodate the diversity of people affected by the institution. Accordingly Habermas notes that in order to live autonomously the private autonomy employed in individual encounters must be complemented by a public autonomy, self-determination of the institutional norms that affect us [30]. It may seem strange at first to classify nosology as an institutional norm, but there can be little debate about the immense public impact of decisions institutionalized in the DSM. These impacts are, of course, felt in terms of forensic issues and insurance reimbursement. But, truthfully, the DSM does a great deal to structure the very nature of the clinical encounter between patient and clinician. The philosopher of science Philip Kitcher [31] has noted more generally that the public impact of science entails a moral prerogative to develop science according to the interests of the citizens impacted by that science. Incorporating patients into the process of developing nosology is a means of assuring that their needs and interests are being addressed. As Sadler and Fulford [32] have noted the potential for patient contributions here is not limited to monitoring for stigmatizing language. It extends all the way down to determining the boundaries between normalcy and disorder. While patients are the preeminent stakeholders in terms of the institutional impact of nosology they have traditionally been the most marginalized in terms of impact upon development of the science. Normative validity entails a more significant role for patients in the development of nosology.

For theoretical purposes it is possible to neatly separate the logic of empirical validity claims from the logic of normative validity claims. In reality, in the practice of science normative and empirical issues are thoroughly intertwined throughout the process. The challenge of integrating patients into the scientific process is that patient needs and interests must be interpreted in the context of scientific contingencies. Nonetheless, the practice of informed consent has already established patients' ability to competently determine their own needs and interests in the context of scientific knowledge. The challenge in shifting to establishing public autonomy as opposed to private autonomy is that the clarification of an individual's interests and needs are not sufficient. As Habermas [33] notes, "Only *generalizable* value-orientations, which all participants (and all those affected) can accept with good reasons as appropriate for regulating the subject matter at hand, and which can thereby acquire binding normative force, pass this threshold." Pioneering work in "user-led research" has begun to explore the process of integrating patient values into the scientific process [34–37]. The complex mixture of epistemic and evaluative elements in the development of nosology underscores the value of integrating scientists who have experienced illness first hand into the process [38].

Concluding Remarks

Elizabeth H. Flanagan, Larry Davidson, and John S. Strauss [39, 40] have emphasized that patient descriptions of illness experiences are an important scientific resource that has been largely neglected in the development of psychiatric nosology to date. Bruce Cuthbert and Thomas Insel [41] are skeptical about the value of this approach because they don't feel that it will help solve the major problems besetting nosology today. They delineate these problems as heterogeneity of the disorders, excessive comorbidity, and the increasingly frequent use of Not Otherwise Specified (NOS) diagnoses. They go on to assert that the neuro-circuitry first and foremost approach of the RDoC project is in a better position to solve these problems. But whether or not comorbidity and heterogeneity really are the foremost problems besetting nosology today is not an empirical question but rather an evaluative and normative question. A syndromal approach to diagnosis is not valuable to medicine solely as a temporary stand-in until a biological etiology is discovered. It is valuable to medicine because it keeps medicine attuned to symptoms that cause distress and therefore to matters of relevance to patients. The fear that the neuro-circuitry first approach of RDoC runs the risk of losing touch with the matters of most relevance to patients is only underscored by a quick dismissal of the value of scientific research into the salient features of illness experience. The leadership of the DSM-5 confidently declared, "Mental disorder syndromes will eventually be redefined to reflect more useful diagnostic categories ('to carve nature at its joints') as well as dimensional discontinuities between disorders and clear thresholds between pathology and normality" [3]. But this assertion stands in stark contrast to the difficulties encountered in categorizing autism, for example, and discriminating between valued aspects of identity and unwanted sources of suffering. The relative value of research into illness experience, and the biological, psychological, and social factors that affect that illness experience are all normative questions. It is not clear that the marginalization of psychosocial research within the science of nosology is justifiable. But, what is clear is that the valid resolution of these normative questions hinges upon a fair process and that a fair process does entail the integration of patient perspectives.

References

1. Regier DA, Kuhl EA, Kupfer DJ, McNulty JP. Patient involvement in the development of DSM-5. Psychiatry. 2010;73(4):308–10.
2. Regier DA. Dimensional approaches to psychiatric classification: refining the research agenda for DSM-5: an introduction. Int J Methods Psychiatr Res. 2007;16 Suppl 1:S1–5. doi:10.1002/mpr.209.
3. Regier DA, Narrow WE, Kuhl EA, Kupfer DJ. The conceptual development of DSM-5. Am J Psychiatry. 2009;166(6):645–50.
4. Decker HS. How Kraepelinian was Kraepelin? How Kraepelinian are the neo-Kraepelinians?—from Emil Kraepelin to DSM-III. Hist Psychiatry. 2007;18(3):337–60. doi:10.1177/0957154X07078976.

5. Spitzer RL. Values and assumptions in the development of DSM-III and DSM-III-R: an insider's perspective and a belated response to Sadler, Hulgus, and Agich's "On values in recent American psychiatric classification". J Nerv Ment Dis. 2001;189(6):351–9.
6. Robins E, Guze SB. Establishment of diagnostic validity in psychiatric illness: its application to schizophrenia. Am J Psychiatry. 1970;126(7):983–7.
7. Murphy D. Philosophy of psychiatry. In: Zalta EN, editor. The stanford encyclopedia of philosophy fall 2010 edition. Available from: http://plato.stanford.edu/archives/fall2010/entries/psychiatry/.
8. Compton WM, Guze SB. The neo-Kraepelinian revolution in psychiatric diagnosis. Eur Arch Psychiatry Clin Neurosci. 1995;245:196–201.
9. Kendell R, Jablensky A. Distinguishing between the validity and utility of psychiatric diagnoses. Am J Psychiatry. 2003;160(1):4–12.
10. Jaspers K. General psychopathology [J. Hoenig and M.W. Hamilton, trans.]. Chicago: University of Chicago Press; 1963.
11. Ghaemi SN. Nosologomania: DSM & Karl Jaspers' critique of Kraepelin. Philoso Ethics Humanit Med. 2009;4(10). doi:10.1186/1747-5341-4-10.
12. Schwartz MA, Wiggins OP. Diagnosis and ideal types: a contribution to psychiatric classification. Compr Psychiatry. 1987;28(4):277–91.
13. Zachar P. The practical kinds model as a pragmatist theory of classification. Philos Psychiatr Psychol. 2002;9(3):219–27.
14. Lewis B. The biopsychosocial model and philosophic pragmatism: is George Engel a pragmatist? Philos Psychiatr Psychol. 2007;14(4):299–310.
15. Kendler KS. Explanatory models for psychiatric illness. Am J Psychiatry. 2008;165:695–702.
16. Kendler KS. Toward a philosophical structure for psychiatry. Am J Psychiatry. 2005;162:433–40.
17. Schaffner KF. Clinical and etiological psychiatric diagnoses: do causes count? In: Kendler JZ, editor. Descriptions & prescriptions: values, mental disorders, and the DSMs. Baltimore: The Johns Hopkins University Press; 2002. p. 271–90.
18. Kendler KS. Toward a scientific psychiatric nosology: strengths and limitations. Arch Gen Psychiatry. 1990;47:969–73.
19. Insel T, Cuthbert B, Garvey M, Heinssen R, Pine DS, Quinn K, et al. Research domain criteria (RDoC): toward a new classification framework for research on mental disorders. Am J Psychiatry. 2010;167(7):748–51.
20. Schwartz MA, Wiggins OP. The hegemony of the DSMs. In: Kendler JZ, editor. Descriptions & prescriptions: values, mental disorders, and the DSMs. Baltimore: The Johns Hopkins University Press; 2002. p. 199–209.
21. Rubin J. Political liberalism and values-based practice: processes above outcomes or rediscovering the priority of the right over the good. Philos Psychiatr Psychol. 2009;15:117–23.
22. Baynes K. The normative grounds of social criticism: Kant, Rawls, and Habermas. Albany: State University of New York Press; 2002.
23. Kant I. Groundwork of the metaphysics of morals [M. Gregor trans. and ed.]. Cambridge: Cambridge University Press; 1998.
24. Habermas J. Moral consciousness and communicative action [C. Lenhardt and S.W. Nicholsen trans.]. Cambridge, Massachusetts: The MIT Press; 1990.
25. Rawls J. A theory of justice. Cambridge, MA: Harvard University Press; 1971.
26. Longino H. Science as social knowledge: values and objectivity in social inquiry. Princeton, NJ: Princeton University Press; 1990.
27. Faden RR, Beauchamp TL. A history and theory of informed consent. New York: Oxford University Press; 1986.
28. Beauchamp TL, McCullough LB. Medical ethics: the moral responsibilities of physicians. Englewood Cliffs, NJ: Prentice-Hall, Inc.; 1984.
29. Pellegrino ED, Thomasma DC. A philosophical basis of medical practice: toward a philosophy and ethic of the healing professions. New York: Oxford University Press; 1981.

30. Habermas J. Between facts and norms: contributions to a discourse theory of law and democracy [W. Rehg trans.]. Cambridge, Massachusetts: The MIT Press; 1996.
31. Kitcher P. Science, truth, and democracy. New York: Oxford University Press; 2001.
32. Sadler JZ, Fulford B. Should patients and their families contribute to the *DSM-5* process? Psychiatr Serv. 2004;55(2):133–8.
33. Habermas J. The inclusion of the other: studies in political theory. Cambridge, MA: The MIT Press; 1998.
34. Faulkner A, Thomas P. User-led research and evidence-based medicine. Br J Psychiatry. 2002;180:1–3.
35. Hanley B, Truesdale A, King A, et al. Involving consumers in designing, conducting, and interpreting randomized controlled trials: questionnaire survey. BMJ. 2001;322:519–23.
36. Perkins R. What constitutes success? The relative priority of service users' and clinicians' views of mental health services. Br J Psychiatry. 2001;179:9–10.
37. Rose D. Collaborative research between users and professionals: peaks and pitfalls. Psychiatr Bull. 2003;27:404–6.
38. Rose D. Having a diagnosis is a qualification for the job. BMJ. 2003;326:1331.
39. Flanagan EH, Davidson L, Strauss JS. Issues for DSM-5: incorporating patients' subjective experiences. Am J Psychiatry. 2007;164(3):391–2.
40. Flanagan EH, Davidson L, Strauss JS. The need for patient-subjective data in the DSM and the ICD. Psychiatry. 2010;73(4):297–307.
41. Cuthbert B, Insel T. The data of diagnosis: new approaches to psychiatric classification. Psychiatry. 2010;73(4):311–4.

Chapter 6
The Paradox of Professional Success: Grand Ambition, Furious Resistance, and the Derailment of the DSM-5 Revision Process

Owen Whooley and Allan V. Horwitz

Future observers of the psychiatric profession might well point to the weekend beginning on May 5, 2012 as the crucial turning point in shaping the DSM-5. From the start, the DSM-5 Task Force viewed the revision process as an opportunity to introduce some radical innovations into psychiatric nosology and perhaps even induce a "paradigm shift" in psychiatry [1]. Initially, their hopes were pinned to the construction of "an etiologically based, scientifically sound classification system" based on genetic and neuroscience research [2]. However, the Task Force quickly realized that this goal was wildly premature. Scraping this path to a paradigm shift, the Task Force settled on dimensionalization as its major innovation. It believed that the introduction of numerical scales would encourage psychiatrists to think about mental disorders as continuous with, rather than distinctly different from, normal behavior and thus resolve the problems brought by the rigid categorical taxonomy of previous DSMs. Dimensional measurement could help psychiatric researchers avoid the reification of diagnostic categories so as to construct research designs more likely to yield valid, biologically based diagnostic categories. Dimensionalization became the central organizing logic behind the revisions and the rallying cry for those trying to reform the profession.

These dimensional aspirations essentially died during the first two weeks of May. First, during the annual meeting of the American Psychiatric Association, the APA assembly voted unanimously to relegate the dimensional scales—the very innovation to which the DSM-5 Work Groups had dedicated years of labor—to the appendix of the DSM-5 for further study. Citing on "undue burden" that the "unproven severity scales" would place on clinicians, the Assembly dashed what

O. Whooley
Department of Sociology, University of New Mexico, Albuquerque, NM, USA
e-mail: owenwho@unm.edu

A.V. Horwitz (✉)
Department of Sociology and Institute for Health, Health Care Policy,
and Aging Research, Rutgers University, New Brunswick, NJ, USA
e-mail: ahorwitz@sas.rutgers.edu

little hope was left for a radical change to the DSM-5 [3]. The same week Allan Frances, Chair of the DSM-IV Task Force, wrote an editorial piece in the *New York Times*, condemning the DSM-5 Task Force. Frances had been carrying out his campaign against the DSM-5 for nearly 3 years, mainly through editorials in professional journals and regular blog postings on the *Psychiatric Times* website. But with the *New York Times* article, the internal debate over DSM-5 become glaringly public. Arguing that the DSM-5 "promises to be a disaster" Frances made the radical suggestion that the sole responsibility for psychiatric nosology should be taken away from the APA and broadened to allow "all mental health disciplines" to have input [4]. Given the DSM's central role in defining the American psychiatric profession, this suggestion signaled a radical departure. It was all the more startling coming from a former chair of the DSM.

Taking a step back from psychiatry's interprofessional squabbling, the rage that surrounds the DSM revision process seems strange. After all, it is only a medical taxonomy. Other taxonomies, like the International Classification of Disease (ICD), hardly register in the popular conscious. They certainly do not warrant front page stories in the *New York Times*. No other professional organization dedicates as much energy and resources into their classificatory systems as the APA. Indeed, the power of classificatory systems stems from their general invisibility; they are inescapably built into our "information environment," dictating standards that we follow but rarely question [5]. Taxonomies are typically mundane and unobtrusive parts of modern life, rarely noticed, much less fought over vehemently in the pages of the popular press. The DSM is the great exception to this rule. Here we have a case in which the identity and authority of psychiatry hinges—or at least internally seems to hinge—on how it structures its taxonomy.

The periodic revisions to the DSM have become ritual moments for the profession to assess itself, and for the DSM-5 Task Force, psychiatry's situation is, if not dire, at least troublesome. Upon first glance, its concerns might seem overwrought, and its ambitious agenda, curious. After all, in the decades following the first "paradigm shift" in the revisions to DSM-III, the manual's influence has grown tremendously. In 1980 the development of the DSM-III shored up the professional prestige of psychiatry by embracing the biomedical model [6–9]. The DSM-III revisions were framed as a necessary, albeit temporary step in the road to situating psychiatry more deeply in medical science. From a professional standpoint they were an unqualified success. The manual has become fully entrenched in all facets of mental health, from research to education, from clinical practice to FDA drug trials, from insurance reimbursement to epidemiological studies. DSM diagnostic codes and criteria are key to getting anything done in the mental health field. Psychiatry literally defines the field of mental health through the DSM [10].

But despite DSM's tremendous influence all is not well in psychiatry. In addition to the typical frustrations under which psychiatrists chafe (e.g. competition from primary care doctors and other mental health professionals, increasing oversight by insurance companies, etc.), the field is undergoing an intellectual crisis born from the persistent elusiveness of any biomarker for mental illness, much less the identification of biological/physiological etiologies for the overwhelming majority of mental illnesses. Two decades after the "Decade of the Brain," the science of mental disorders remains in its infancy. Faced with this validity crisis, the Task Force identified the DSM's categorical system of classifying mental disorders as the culprit; its "serious flaws have become increasingly problematic for research and clinical use" [11]. In an attempt to repeat history, psychiatry's strategy to address its intellectual crisis is the same—fix the taxonomic system, fix psychiatry. But as the Assembly's rejection of dimensionalization shows, times have changed, and conditions today are such that pulling off a feat similar to DSM-III has proven difficult, if not impossible.

This chapter embeds the current controversy over DSM-5 within the professional politics of American psychiatry over the last three decades. Undergirding the relatively arcane struggle over dimensionalization are questions about the direction of the psychiatric profession and its future prospects. An occupation can be said to be a profession when it has assumed a dominant position in the division of labor so that it "gains control over the determination of the substance of its own work" [12]. In contrast with the logic of the free market, professions are based on the logic of monopolies granted on the understanding that the particular tasks a profession performs are "so different from those of most workers that self-control is essential" [13]. To wield expertise effectively and safely, professionals therefore must dictate the nature of their work without outside meddling.

The allocation of professional authority evolves according to interprofessional competition. Professions exist within an ecological system, in which different professions struggle over jurisdictions of work in what is largely a zero-sum game [14]. The drive for autonomy and authority leads professions into conflict with one another and make their histories interdependent, as competition with other professions shapes the organizational structure and strategies adopted by any particular profession. In claiming a jurisdiction professions ask society to recognize its cognitive structure by granting exclusive rights to control and dictate the nature of their own work. Knowledge, therefore, is the "currency of competition" among professions, as definition of reality and the production of knowledge are central to the ability of a profession to gain control over a jurisdiction, to claim expertise and in turn, authority [4]. Professions must convince other actors that they possess special expertise—and that their knowledge is unavailable and/or inaccessible to just anyone—in order to attain cultural authority and special privileges in the form of market protections [13, 15].

To make sense of the very public debates over DSM-5, we examine the DSM through the lens of professional politics, situating psychiatry within the larger field of mental health. It is out of competition with other mental health professionals that psychiatry's most curious idiosyncrasy—its dependence on a taxonomy for its authority—is explicable. The DSM has become *the* means by which the profession has dealt with crisis and shored up its jurisdiction. In many ways, the recent history of the American psychiatric profession, its triumphs and failures, *is* the history of the DSM. In the late 1970s, the profession was besieged as its intellectual energy waned under the intellectually enervated psychoanalytic model. In 1980, Robert Spitzer essentially transformed what was a document largely incidental to professional practice into the final word on defining both the universe of mental disorders and the identity of psychiatry itself. Now, faced with another professional crisis borne from real and troubling uncertainties in psychiatric knowledge, the DSM-5 Task Force is essentially attempting to repeat history, that is, to shore up psychiatry's jurisdiction and status within the mental health field by carrying out another radical revision. Thus, this ostensibly drab document contains within its codes and categories the fascinating story of how psychiatry has tried to secure its professional jurisdiction in lieu of biomarkers for mental illness.

Only by acknowledging the tremendous professional stakes of the DSM, can we make sense of the intensity of the debates over dimensionality and account for the failure of the Task Force to achieve a radical paradigm shift. Given that psychiatry has built its legitimacy on the DSM, it cannot completely repudiate its underlying logic, lest it forfeit its current legitimacy. The very success of the first DSM paradigm shift complicates the professional politics involved in the revision by foreclosing radical change. However, the built-in inertia in the revision process stifles intellectual innovation and threatens intellectual stagnation for the profession. The DSM-5 revision process has opened the door to questions about the future of psychiatry but the polarizing debate it has caused has left the profession handcuffed, unable to pursue any answers.

The DSM-III Revolution

Psychoanalytic and psychodynamic perspectives on mental disorders were the primary influence on the DSM-I and DSM-II. These perspectives viewed mental disorders as continuous with, rather than discrete from, normal behavior. Because there were no firm lines to be drawn between the ill and the well, diagnosis—and the careful delineation of disorders that could facilitate accurate diagnoses—was not an essential part of psychiatric practice. The early editions of the DSM served modest administrative purposes, but were generally ignored by psychiatrists [16].

However, beginning in the 1960s and extending into the 1970s, psychiatry experienced a crisis that called into question its legitimacy and that would eventually lead reformers to elevate the DSM to great importance. In the 1960s American psychiatry was still largely committed to psychoanalysis. This commitment, however, weakened in the face of a number of challenges, including the emergence of other mental health professions that offered alternative therapies to psychoanalysis, social scientific research that exposed the inconsistency and arbitrariness of psychiatric diagnosis [17, 18], and an anti-psychiatry movement that popularized dehumanizing depictions of the profession [19, 20]. Critics questioned whether mental illnesses were real and, in turn, whether psychiatrists served any positive purpose. An extremely bitter and very public debate over the diagnosis of homosexuality as a mental illness further fueled such critiques by undermining the scientific bona fides of the profession [21]. In addition to these problems, psychiatry suffered an organizational blow when the passage of the Community Mental Health Act in 1963 led to the widespread deinstitutionalization of mental patients, putting the final nail in the coffin of what was once the institutional stronghold of psychiatric power [22].

By the late 1970s the confluence of these multiple critiques compromised the credibility of psychiatry. The task force charged with developing the DSM-III, under the direction of Robert Spitzer, interpreted these crises as deriving from a single intellectual problem—a lack of reliability in diagnoses. Limited reliability led to inconsistency in defining mental illnesses, wrongful institutionalization of patients, inability to conduct multisite research, and hostile public views of psychiatry. The DSM-III Task Force's primary goal became to radically remake the classificatory system of mental disorders in order to achieve better reliability. In the process, it ushered in a sweeping paradigm shift in psychiatry.

The revisions to the DSM-III sought to increase reliability through moving psychiatry away from the fluid psychoanalytic understanding of mental illness toward a standardized nosology of fixed disease categories. They overthrew the broad, continuous, and vague concepts of dynamic psychiatry and replaced them with a discrete system of classification that treated mental disorders as discrete diseases. This nosology rigorously segregated the pathological from the normal, in a way that the previous psychodynamic model never did.

Organizing diagnostic categories according to symptom clusters, the revisions de-emphasized broad concepts such as neuroses and personality in order to put psychiatry on firmer scientific grounds and root it within medicine. According to Spitzer, "The manual's [DSM] real significance is that it shows psychiatry becoming more of a science. The criteria for making a diagnosis are spelled out with great specificity, and patients will benefit because the diagnoses have treatment implications," [quoted in 23]. While the DSM-III revisions were advertised as agnostic toward different theoretical schools of psychiatry [24], the entire endeavor—delineating discrete disease categories to facilitate diagnostic consistency—implied an endorsement of the biomedical model. The revisions were sold as ways to improve treatment through empirically based research programs and targeted diagnoses. The new paradigm of diagnostic psychiatry organized symptoms into discrete disease entities with the expectation that the organic bases of these entities would soon be discovered [6]. In other words, the revisions to the DSM were a strategy to attain a biomedical model by understanding illnesses as stable entities that can be explained in terms of specific causal mechanisms located in the brain. The hope was that the identification of the elusive biological or genetic markers for mental disorders would follow from the standardized classification system. DSM-III promised a future when specific etiologies were discovered for specific disorders and, in turn, specific treatments would emerge.

By professional standards the revisions were unimaginably successful. Gerald Klerman, the highest ranking government psychiatrist, framed the revisions as a "reaffirmation on the part of American psychiatry to its medical identity and its commitment to scientific medicine" [7]. The DSM-III allowed psychiatry to align itself more firmly with scientific medicine and thus to justify psychiatry's trump card in the ecology of mental health professions—the sole right to prescribe drugs. The DSM-III and its subsequent editions (DSM-III-R, DSM-IV, and DSM-IV-TR) monopolized diagnosis not only in psychiatry, but in the field of mental health more generally. The widespread adoption of DSM categories by clinicians, researchers, insurance companies, pharmaceutical manufacturers, and other mental health professions validated psychiatry's claim to special expertise. By the 1990s psychiatry had solidified its position in a mental health market that was becoming increasingly medicalized.

In an important sense, then, DSM-III and its subsequent editions, served an essential promissory function in that they were framed as providing the foundation for future breakthroughs in psychiatry [25]. With a common language, reliable categories, and a well-defined universe of objects of analyses, psychiatrists would be able to secure the causal knowledge and therapeutic effectiveness that had long eluded the profession. DSM-III would be the bridge to making psychiatry scientific. As long as the DSM-III and its promises were accepted, psychiatry's standing within the mental health profession was safe.

The New Crisis of Validity

Because the DSM has been so successful, it can be difficult to see the precarious trends that psychiatry is currently experiencing. As psychiatry has become more integrated into medicine, its services have increasingly been reduced to drug management and treatment. For the most part, psychiatrists maintain sole control of prescribing drugs but they have largely ceded the practice of psychotherapy to other mental health professionals. The percentage of visits to psychiatrists that included psychotherapy dropped from 44 % in 1996–1997 to 29 % in 2004–2005 [26]. Grounding their expertise in drug management distinguishes psychiatrists from other mental health professionals but also puts them into competition with other doctors. General practitioners write most prescriptions for psychopharmaceutical drugs [27]. Furthermore, the DSM diagnoses do not guide prescribing practice; most psychoactive drugs work across diagnostic categories [28, 29]. In adopting a distinctively medical identity, psychiatrists both narrowed the scope of their special expertise vis-à-vis other mental health workers and came into professional conflict with other physicians. In addition, critiques over the medicalization of mental disorders—ranging from social science research [30] to conspiratorial accusations by scientologists—although perhaps not as dire, echo the legitimacy crisis of the 1970s. But whereas the reliability problems drove the 1970s crisis, problems of validity are at the heart of psychiatry's precarious professional situation at present. The DSM-III's promise that reliability would lead to validity has not been realized.

The problem of validity is not a new one for psychiatry. The entire history of the field's professional insecurity—its ever-present concern over maintaining its jurisdiction—is driven by a frustratingly persistent fact: no one has ever found a dependable biological marker for a mental disorder. Nor has it discovered the etiology of mental disorders. This places psychiatry in a curious position vis-à-vis its claims to medical science. The question of how to define valid cases of mental disorder has perennially bedeviled psychiatry. As historian Gerald Grob [31] points out, every generation has "insisted that the specialty stood on the threshold of fundamental breakthroughs that would revolutionize the ways in which mental disorders were understood and treated... Many etiological theories (hereditarian, Freudian, neurochemical, etc.) have been proposed to great fanfare only to buckle under the weight of their initial promise. In other branches of medicine, by contrast, the demonstration of a relationship between the presence of certain symptoms and a specific bacterial organism had led to the development of a new classification system based on etiology rather than symptomatology. The inability to pursue a parallel course left psychiatry with a classification system based on external symptoms that tended to vary in the extreme." DSM-III alleviated some of this insecurity by promising that reliable categories would eventually yield valid ones. As long as this assurance was accepted, psychiatry's position within the ecology of mental health professions was secure.

Three decades after the paradigm shift to diagnostic psychiatry, the DSM's scientific accomplishments have not met its initial promises. This underlying concern that reliability has not promoted advances in knowledge drove the Task Force to attempt a new paradigm shift, one that ostensibly targets validity. As the DSM-5 Task Force observes, "In the more than 30 years since the introduction of the Feighner criteria by Robins and Guze, which eventually led to DSM-III, the goal of validating these syndromes and discovering common etiologies has remained elusive" [2].

In general, there is a growing concern that the DSM-III model is "more likely to obscure than to elucidate research findings" [2]. Put succinctly, "the reliance on categorical diagnoses in past research studies may be a major factor in how little we yet know of the causes and cures of mental disorders" [32]. The problems with the DSM-III model, according to this line of thinking, are threefold. First, the DSM categories do not reflect discrete entities. This is evident in the high rates of comorbidity across categories, which, according to the Task Force, corrupts research [2]. How can specific remedies be discovered if disease categories that underlie research overlap? Moreover, psychiatrists often rely on the "Not-otherwise-specified" (NOS) diagnostic category [33], suggesting the inadequacies of the current definitions. A second concern is that by drawing arbitrary boundaries between categories, psychiatric research could be entirely misdirected, searching for phantoms. Finally, the key factor driving the proposed paradigm shift to DSM-5 is that the binary logic of DSM-III (either one has a mental disorder or not) may not be sensitive enough to detect genetic variance. The bluntness of DSM categories may obscure the ways in which genetic variance becomes manifest, and therefore prevent etiological discoveries. These problems have led to a situation in which "psychiatry is at a crossroads with DSM-V" [34]. And once again psychiatry has turned to the DSM to overcome stagnation in psychiatric knowledge and to shore up its jurisdictional claims.

Dreaming of Dimensions

The DSM-5 Task Force proposed to solve the validity issue by shifting toward a more dimensional conceptualization of mental disorders. Dimensionality may seem like a strange choice for a "new" paradigm shift, because conceiving of mental disorders on a spectrum harkens back to the psychoanalytic tradition that the profession had spent decades shedding. Unlike the psychoanalytic tradition, however, this new dimensionality is rooted in quantification.

Since DSM-III, every edition of the DSM has classified mental disorders as discrete categorical syndromes. Mental illness categories were constructed as clusters of symptom manifestations. In order to meet a diagnosis, a given patient would have to demonstrate a certain numbers of symptoms within the syndrome. Categories are organized around an either/or logic: if a patient meets the proposed criteria, she is seen as having a clinically significant psychiatric diagnosis; if not, the patient is not seen as having mental disorder. For example, the category of major depressive disorder (MDD) contains a list of nine symptoms. To meet the threshold for the diagnosis of MDD, a patient would have to demonstrate at least five of the nine listed symptoms. Patients with four or fewer symptoms cannot receive this diagnosis.

Dimensionalization changes this logic. Rather than viewing disease categories as categorically different from normal states, dimensions represent mental illness and well-being as existing on a spectrum. Patients would be assessed along a continuum and diagnoses would expressed numerically. Mental disorders, formerly conceived as *qualitatively different*, would now be construed as only quantitatively different from normality. Were the DSM-5 to embody this proposal, psychiatric nosology would feature a new logic of classification in which the pathological differs in magnitude, not in kind, from the normal.

The Task Force's project of dimensionalization involved quantifying mental illness by introducing two types of dimensional scales. First, it would include some overall, cross-cutting dimensional scale to screen all perspective patients. This would yield numerical information on the state of the patient but delay pigeonholing a patient into a specific diagnosis. Rather than restrict assessment to the system of categories, the cross-cutting scale would examine broad biobehavioral symptoms that blur with one another and with normality. This dimensional measure would serve as an important screening device that could facilitate early identification and intervention. After this initial, cross-cutting screening, psychiatrists would derive a diagnosis from an interview in which they would draw on both the initial screen and the diagnostic category. Once they determine a specific diagnosis, the second dimensional intervention would come into play. This would involve using severity scales for each specific disorder in the manual. A patient would receive a numerical ranking of severity for a diagnosis as well as an either/or diagnosis. In order to tailor each severity scale to the specific disease, each work group was granted flexibility to determine how to structure their scales. Some groups quantified particular symptoms and added them up for a composite severity score; others constructed severity scales by simply counting the number of symptom criteria a patient meets. The irony of this flexibility is that it undermines the standardization hard won by DSM-III through promoting divergent diagnostic processes.

Whatever trade-offs with standardization the new scales might have to make, because the current professional malaise has been interpreted a stemming from a problem of validity, the Task Force continued to promote dimensionality. According to their view, dimensionalization has a number of benefits, including: the accumulation of more data beyond binary categories; the facilitation of genetic research by characterizing phenotypic variability more precisely and by increasing potential statistical power without having to increase the size of the study sample [32]; and obtaining the requisite sensitivity to identify of subthreshold conditions that might respond well to interventions.

The diagnostic scales would encourage psychiatrists to conceptualize the patient's ailment in numerical terms. The patient would no longer have MDD but MDD with a specific numerical value attached to it. Herein lies the paradigm-shifting element of these revisions. While various constraints have prevented the DSM-5 Task Force from scrapping the categorical model altogether—the numerical scales bookend the traditional categories—it hoped that the introducing dimensionality into the DSM would foster a revolution in the conception of mental disorders.

Diagnostic Inertia

The potentially radical implications of dimensionality fostered an intense debate among psychiatrists over what are seemingly benign, straightforward, and perhaps even banal scales. Indeed, the DSM-5 revision has created and exacerbated internal tensions within psychiatry that threaten to undermine the exulted status of the DSM. The debate has pitted the DSM-5 Task Force against members of previous task forces. Robert Spitzer and Allen Frances, chairs of the DSM-III and DSM-IV Task Forces, respectively, have been the most ardent critics of the DSM-5 process. The intense debate among research psychiatrists has filtered down to the rank and file and, as psychiatrists choose sides, the unity of the profession has been endangered.

The opponents' criticisms of the DSM-5 are wide-ranging, focusing both on processual and substantive issues. Their major concerns are that the revisions (1) have lacked transparency[1]; (2) have been marred by disorganization, reflected in continuous delays; (3) do not pay due attention to the clinical utility of its proposed changes; (4) proposes new problematic diagnoses (i.e. attenuated psychosis syndrome) without sufficient scientific justification; (5) exacerbate the problem of false

---

[1] Robert Spitzer has focused his criticisms on the lack of transparency in the DSM-5 process, an ironic criticism coming from a man who, by his own admission, controlled every facet of the DSM-III process, and who himself, was repeatedly lambasted for the close nature of his revision process.

positives by lowering the criteria thresholds for a number of diagnostic categories; and (6) introduce untested and unproven dimensional assessment tools when the process lacks the capacity to create such tools. At the core of all these criticisms is a sense that the Task Force, in trying for a paradigm shift, is acting too rashly and opening the profession to unintended consequence and public scorn that will inevitably follow such consequences [35]. The concern with the inclusion of dimensional scales is that "introducing a botched dimensional system prematurely into DSM-V may have the negative effect of poisoning the well for their future acceptance by clinicians…" [36]. The premature actions of the Task Force risk turning the DSM from what is perceived to be a comprehensive and authoritative manual into something that will be subject to constant and radical revisions.

Allan Frances has been the most vocal critic of the proposed changes, waging an unrelenting campaign against the revisions. In editorials in psychiatric journals and his recurrent blog on the *Psychiatric Times* webpage, Frances has taken the DSM-5 Task Force to task for what he sees as hubris and overreach. The unrealistic nature of this premature push for revisions is particularly evident in the dimensional proposals, which he deems the "totally unrealistic ambition to provide diagnostic rating scales for each section of DSM5" [37]. For proprietary reasons the Task Force cannot use preexisting scales,[2] so it has had to develop entirely new ones to include in DSM-5. Frances notes:

> It takes years of painstaking iterative work to develop and test a rating scale. The performance characteristics of each of the candidate items have to be tested. The items then have to be revised, tested again, and revised again, and so on until there is confidence that the scale does indeed measure what it is supposed to measure. The testing must be performed in large and representative samples that include those comparison groups most likely to be confused in the differential diagnosis. The scales must also be tested in primary care settings where so many people are diagnosed and treated with psychotropic medication. [37]

Such a task, according to Frances, is beyond the capacities of the committee. And it is woefully misguided because scientific developments do not justify the push for dimensionality.

The debate has devolved into *ad hominem* attacks. Frances accuses the Task Force of vanity. The Task Force in turn accuses Frances of being disingenuous, conjuring up controversy out of crass economic interests (i.e. possible lost royalties from DSM-IV once the manual is revised) [38]. The rancor has found its way into the DSM-5 work groups. In March, 2009, Jane Costello resigned from the Child and Adolescent Disorders workgroup, circulating a resignation letter in which she expressed that she was "increasingly uncomfortable with the whole underlying principle of rewriting the entire psychiatric taxonomy at one time. I am not aware of any other branch of medicine that does anything like this" [39]. She cited the dimensional proposals as the tipping point that precipitated her resignation, because of the

---

[2]The exception is the PHQ9, a self-reported depression scale sponsored by Pfizer, but now in the public domain.

"possibility of doing a psychometrically careful and responsible job given the time and resources available is remote, while to do anything less is irresponsible" [39]. Others, like Howard Moss, a Task Force member, and John Livesley and Roel Verheul, prominent members of the Personality Disorders Work Group, have resigned as well, publicly condemning the process as they did so [40].

Despite this vitriol, all the disputants seem to agree that a categorical model of mental illness is problematic and that it is more accurate to think of mental illness in dimensional terms. In addition, none dispute that "the difficulty at this moment in history is that many of the problems are coming into clearer focus but the scientific data needed to develop a fully adequate diagnostic system are lacking" [41]. The controversy hinges less on philosophical and more on processual grounds. The question is what to do about this state of affairs *at this moment.* Is the time right for a "paradigm shift"? And if it is, how it can be accomplished with the least amount of disruption? The Task Force, impatient with the status quo and urgent to encourage new directions, has proposed dimensionality, which entails drastic changes to the structure and underlying model of mental illness that the manual promotes. Frances and Spitzer argue for a more conservative approach, keeping the current system in place while building the requisite research and science to justify such changes to the DSM. Recalling his own experiences with the unintended consequences of making changes, Frances wants to err on the side of caution: "Fiddling needlessly with the labels will not advance science and may actually do more harm than good in its effect on clinical care" [42]. Similarly Michael First, text editor of DSM-IV-TR, notes.

> We know that the system we have now doesn't map onto reality, but since we don't what reality is, we have no idea what the paradigm shift might be. Eventually the paradigm shift will reveal itself by the science. That's the way paradigm shifts usually work. The reason why it's difficult to prognosticate that is God knows when that might happen? *Eventually* it's probably going to happen, and *eventually* the current system will become so obviously not viable compared to what we now know, then there will have to be a paradigm shift.[3]

Ironically, part of the problem stems from the sheer success of previous editions of the DSM. The widespread institutionalization of the manual in all facets of the mental health system has translated into great inertia when it comes to altering the manual. Its penetration into all facets of the workaday world of psychiatry makes any changes beyond those at the margin, potentially systemically disruptive. Michael First outlines these potential disruptions: "Adopting a dimensional approach would likely complicate medical record keeping, create administrative and clinical barriers between mental disorders and medical conditions, require a massive retreating effort, disrupt research efforts (e.g., meta-analyses), and complicate clinicians' efforts to integrate prior clinical research using *DSM* categories into clinical practice" [43]. The entire paperwork edifice of psychiatry—from hospital admissions

---

[3] Quote taken from author interview of Michael First, conducted on December 8, 2010, New York, NY.

procedures to insurance reimbursement—would require changes. Reconciling the new system with past research would also be challenging, and perhaps might jeopardize meta-analyses and longitudinal studies. New structured psychiatric interviews protocols would have to be created to address criterion changes. And, clinicians would have to learn these new protocols and figure out how to incorporate scales into their practices.

The Revolution Will Not Materialize

For a profession long sensitive to external criticisms and concerned about its image, the microscope under which the revision process has been placed and the public display of internal discord is disconcerting. The opposition to the revision process caught the attention of the APA's Board of Trustees and in the winter of 2010, they established a Scientific Review Committee charged with assessing the scientific justification of all proposed changes to the DSM. This extra layer of oversight seriously retarded both the pace and possibility of radical changes. Unlike the Work Groups, which can take into account a host of factors when making revisions, including not only scientific evidence but also clinical utility, expert consensus, and practical considerations, the Scientific Review Committee is limited to using research evidence in assessing the changes. This higher standard makes changes more difficult. Moreover, the demand that any changes have sufficient research backing makes it extremely hard to introduce any substantial innovations because the bulk of the psychiatric research is built upon the very DSM categories that the revisers are trying to change. Because DSM categories penetrate psychiatric research designs in such a fundamental way, it is hard to find research supporting alternatives to the categorical model. Thus, for opponents of paradigm shift, the establishment of the Scientific Review Committee was a major win, as its whole rationale is premised on a more iterative understanding of scientific progress.

Despite years of work and the investment of a tremendous amount of resources, it appears that the Task Force's dream of a paradigm shift will not be realized. While Frances and his peers have convinced the APA to reject what they perceive to be the more egregious diagnostic categories—like Psychosis Risk Syndrome—and have effectively constructed barriers to the more radical changes, it is clinicians who seem to have dealt the death knell to dimensionality. Primarily, the public controversy over DSM-5 has involved research psychiatrists, who dominate the DSM revision process. Clinicians, who are the ones who actually have to use the DSM in practice, were largely silent during the early years of the revisions. Indeed, over the course of the debate, both sides—pro-revisionists and critics—have marshaled clinicians to defend their positions, claiming that scales would help clinical practice or that clinicians have never clamored for scales, respectively. But neither side made much of an attempt to actually investigate the wishes of clinicians. Instead they became a cipher onto which each side painted their own preferences.

However, as the process progressed toward its climax, clinicians began to speak up. First, nonpsychiatric professional groups raised concerns. In June 2011, the British Psychological Society [44] circulated a letter that, while largely supportive of dimensionality, condemned the DSM's medicalization of patients' "natural and normal responses to their experiences." This was followed by letters from the Society for Humanistic Psychology, a Division of American Psychological Association [45] and American Counseling Association [46], which echoed psychologists' criticisms of DSM for the last three decades. But clinicians also voiced concern over the proposed dimensional scales: The American Counseling Association [46] stated that while "members were initially supportive of the idea of using dimensional and cross-cutting assessments, but our review of the proposed assessments on the DSM-5 website causes us considerable worry. Little information regarding scale development has been provided and, according to the field trial protocols, there is no evaluation using external validators." The Task Force and the APA formally responded to these critiques but in doing so, largely dismissed their concerns. But when the APA's own membership spoke the APA could no longer ignore the clinical critique.

At the annual meeting of the American Psychiatric Association in May 2012, the APA Assembly voted unanimously to place all the dimensional scales in the appendix of the manual. The rationale for such a dramatic decision was based on the excess burden the scales would place on clinicians. If put in the text, the scales would become the standard of care, and it would be likely that institutions (e.g. hospitals, insurance companies, etc.) would demand that clinicians use them. Given that there has been almost no research showing the practical utility of the scales, the Assembly [3] voted for caution, arguing that the "unproven severity scales" needed more testing. While the vote is not binding, it is extremely unlikely that the APA would ignore it. The Assembly effectively rejected the Task Force's major innovation to DSM-5.

While the Assembly motion addressed severity scales specifically, it also manifested the long standing tension within the profession between clinicians and researchers. Since 1980, psychiatric researchers have primarily written the DSM, and clinicians have long complained about its standardizing, cook-book tendencies. In attempting to homogenize diagnostic practice, the DSM impinges on clinicians' discretion. Before the DSM-III, American psychiatry had a long hermeneutic tradition rooted in individual psychiatrists' nuanced ability to decipher the complexity of individual minds so as to assuage distress. The DSM-III revolution that standardized diagnoses, undermined clinical discretion to a large degree, and clinicians responded with various workarounds to carve a space for autonomy in practice [10, 47]. Quantifying diagnoses would further this de-emphasis of clinical judgment. Consequently, clinicians find themselves in a complicated relationship with the DSM—complications that dimensionality would exacerbate. On the one hand, as members of a profession, psychiatrists gain credibility from the DSM. And insofar as dimensionality would improve scientific research (an issue that is by no means resolved), it could help solidify the prestige of psychiatry. On the other hand, the more that the needs of researchers dictate the DSM and impinge on clinical practice, the more clinical intuition and expertise is devalued. This becomes evident when we consider that one of the major goals of including scales is to *reduce* the need for clinical judgment in diagnosis. Scales may obtain more advanced statistical analyses and knowledge but they do so at the expense of clinical intuition. In rejecting the severity scales the Assembly not only squashed all talk of paradigm shift; it also struck a blow for clinical discretion.

Given these tensions, and given the fact that the DSM is morphing into something inadequate to the tasks of both researchers and clinicians, one has to wonder if decoupling the two endeavors—research and clinical practice—might be the better way to go. Michael First raised just this point, arguing that the end result of these struggles is "a lowest common denominator that creates problems" for everyone.[4] If dimensional scales are watered down to meet the demand of clinicians then they no longer will accomplish their research goals. If clinicians *still* find the watered down scales too cumbersome and ignore them, then the entire revision process would be a no-win situation that leaves in its wake little more than angered, disaffected factions. Indeed, this sentiment is driving a new NIMH initiative called the Research Domain Criterion (RDoC) that seeks to create a new dimensional taxonomy, based on dimensions of observable behavior and neurobiological measures, for research purposes only. Eventually it is hoped that this new taxonomy, which draws upon the latest research in genomics, pathophysiology, neuroscience, and behavioral science, will be more useful for researchers and will lead to that elusive holy grail. Unburdened by the constraints of making such a system useful in clinical practice, RDoC promises to allow psychiatric researchers to pursue their own goals. Thus, for many researchers, RDoC has absorbed the hope for paradigm shift with which the DSM revision process began. As RDoC is an NIMH initiative, it remains to be seen how it will affect the APA's professional agenda. Given the extent to which the APA has depended on its taxonomic activities to justify its professional authority, what would happen to such authority if this responsibility was taken away from the psychiatric profession?

Conclusion

The dreams of a paradigm shift that motivated the DSM-5 revision process have largely been discarded. The Task Force, scrambling to meet its May 2013 deadline, has little time to address the Assembly motion. In an attempt to save face, it is now proffering the notion that the DSM will become a "living document"—rather than having a periodic wholesale revision the manual will be revised incrementally as needs arise—as the true innovation. But given that the details of how this would be

---

[4] Quote taken from author interview of Michael First, conducted on December 8, 2010, New York, NY.

achieved have not been laid out, it is clear that the promotion of the idea of a "living document" represents little more than the Task Force trying to whitewash what has been a disastrous process.

So what can we expect from the DSM-5? First, despite all its problems, the manual will likely be a financial success. Although the actual text might not represent much of a change and/or improvement over DSM-IV, because the DSM has become so central to mental health practice people will buy it. But they will not be buying a game changing document. The grouping of some disorders is slated to change, as will criteria for specific categories. But there is no revolution here. The categorical system will remain intact, although the text of some of the definitions will incorporate more dimensional language. Only time will tell whether the perennial concerns with the DSM—overmedicalization, diagnostic expansion, and proliferation of disorders—will worsen or improve in the new manual.

Whatever the final product looks like, the manual's status as a source of professional prestige has been compromised. While it is far too early to assess the implications of the public debate, the Assembly's retreat and the internal bad blood that the process has created have damaged psychiatry's professional standing. We seem to be witnessing the limits of the strategy of shoring up professional jurisdiction through taxonomic revisions. The DSM-5 tried, but failed, to repeat Spitzer's feat. Certainly the lessons from this revision will make future task forces (if there are any) squeamish in trying to use the DSM to achieve paradigm shift.

The DSM purports to be many different things at once. According to the DSM-IV-TR [48]:

> The utility and credibility of DSM-IV require that it focus on its clinical, research, and educational purposes and be supported by an extensive empirical foundation. *Our highest priority has been to provide a helpful guide to clinical practice.* We hoped to make DSM-IV practical and useful for clinicians by striving for brevity of criteria sets, clarity of language, and explicit statements of the constructs embodied in the diagnostic criteria. An additional goal was to facilitate research and improve communication among clinicians and researchers. We were also mindful of the use of DSM-IV for improving the collection of clinical information and as an educational tool for teaching psychopathology (emphasis added).

In addition to these clinical, research, and educational goals, the manual is also "fundamental to medical record keeping" [48], "a necessary tool for collecting and communicating accurate public health statistics" [48], an authoritative text for legal purposes, and is incorporated into the bureaucratic morass of the U.S. health insurance system. Moreover, it is meant to be useful, and used, by "clinicians with different orientations, among many different professionals, across different practice settings" [48]. Given the sheer scope and diversity of its avowed mandate, the past success of the DSM is all the more impressive. That it became the vehicle that re-legitimated psychiatry is one of the intellectual marvels of the twentieth century.

But one wonders if the DSM can continue to bear the weight of these competing interests, if the center can hold. The debates over dimensionality have intensified and highlighted the inherent problems of hitching so many demands to a single document. Internal disputes among the psychiatric research community over what intellectual agendas to push and how fast to push them have always existed.

But given the DSM's diffuse and widespread influence, any occasion to promote a particular agenda *through* the manual creates incredibly high stakes. These stakes might not be specific to dimensionality—any dramatic change proposed would likely face similar resistance—but the line has been drawn to oppose other candidates for paradigm change as too premature or undeveloped.

In many ways, the strategy Spitzer and the DSM-III Task Force adopted fit the needs of the profession at the time. Insofar as the crises of the 1960s and 1970s reflected reliability problems and inconsistent use of diagnostic terms, the DSM-III brought a measure of coherence to a reeling profession by defining the universe of mental illness and providing a common language for psychiatry. And because the DSM was not central to the profession at the time of the revision, Spitzer was given free rein to edit as he saw fit. His revisions bolstered psychiatry's legitimacy, while buying it time until the science caught up. Such promissory practices served a legitimizing function, allowing psychiatry to deflect criticism by pointing to a brighter, more enlightened future. Times have changed as has the profession. Because the DSM saturates the mental health field and forms the core of psychiatry's identity, it has become nearly impossible to introduce radical changes. The professional stakes of the document have simply become too high to allow for anything other than tinkering around the edges. Despite the Task Force's dogged dedication to doing something dramatic—and the time and resources that backed these goals—DSM-5 is slated to look a lot like DSM-IV.

Eventually, only scientific findings can produce the breakthroughs the DSM-5 Task Force wanted to accomplish. No science, medical or otherwise, can justify itself solely on nosology. Paradigm shifts cannot occur via fiat alone. Even the DSM-III, despite its successes, failed to achieve its lofty aspirations. The science must be there. Psychiatry's persistent, vexing problem is that its scientific base, its foundation of knowledge, lacks the track record of discoveries found in other medical fields. In lieu of this, the profession has attempted to shore up its jurisdiction through the DSM, at least buying time until a true paradigm shift is realized or the "holy grail" is found. But the fate of the DSM-5 shows the limitations of garnering scientific legitimacy through a nosology.

References

1. Regier DA, Kupfer DJ. DSM-V forum: progress in research and development. Paper presented at the annual meeting of American Psychiatric Association, San Francisco, CA; 2009.
2. Kupfer DJ, First MB, Regier DA, editors. A research agenda for DSM-V. Washington, DC: American Psychiatric; 2002.
3. Assembly of the American Psychiatric Association. Motion on crosscutting dimensions and severity scales. Passed at the annual meeting of American Psychiatric Association, New York, NY; 2012.
4. Frances A. Diagnosing the DSM. The New York Times. 11 May 2012;19.
5. Bowker GC, Star SL. Sorting things out: classification and its consequences. Cambridge, MA: MIT; 1999.

6. Horwitz AV. Creating mental illness. Chicago: University of Chicago Press; 2002.
7. Kirk S, Kutchins H. The selling of DSM: the rhetoric of science in psychiatry. Piscataway, NJ: Aldine; 1992.
8. Klerman G. The significance of DSM–III in American Psychiatry. In: Spitzer R, Williams J, Skodol A, editors. International perspectives on DSM-III. Washington, DC: American Psychiatric Press; 1983.
9. Young A. The harmony of illusions: inventing post-traumatic stress disorder. Princeton, NJ: Princeton University Press; 1995.
10. Whooley O. Diagnostic ambivalence: psychiatric workarounds and the Diagnostic and Statistical Manual of Mental Disorders. Sociol Health Illn. 2010;32(3):452–69.
11. Cuthbert BN. Dimensional models of psychopathology: research agenda and clinical utility. J Abnorm Psychol. 2005;114(4):565–9.
12. Freidson E. Professional dominance: the social structure of medical care. New York: Atherton; 1970.
13. Freidson E. Professionalism: the third logic. Chicago: University of Chicago Press; 2001.
14. Abbott A. The system of professions: an essay on the division of expert labor. Chicago: University of Chicago Press; 1988.
15. Starr P. The social transformation of American medicine. New York: Basic Books; 1982.
16. Grob GN. Origins of DSM-I: a study in appearance and reality. Am J Psychiatry. 1991; 148(4):421–31.
17. Kendell R, Cooper J, Gourlay A, Copeland J, Sharpe L, Gurland B. Diagnostic criteria of American and British psychiatrists. Arch Gen Psychiatry. 1971;25(2):123.
18. Rosenhan D. On being sane in insane places. Science. 1973;179(4070):250.
19. Laing RD. The divided self; a study of sanity and madness. London: Tavistock; 1960.
20. Szasz TS. The myth of mental illness; foundations of a theory of personal conduct. New York: Hoeber-Harper; 1961.
21. Bayer R. Homosexuality and American psychiatry: the politics of diagnosis. Princeton, NJ: Princeton University Press; 1987.
22. Grob GN. From asylum to community: mental health policy in modern America. Princeton: University Press; 1991.
23. Sobel D. New psychiatric definitions expected to affect therapy. The New York Times. 11 Dec 1971;C1.
24. American Psychiatric Association. Diagnostic and statistical manual of mental disorders: DSM-III. Washington, DC: American Psychiatric; 1980.
25. Fortun M. Promising genomics: Iceland and deCODE genetics in a world of speculation. Berkeley, CA: University of California Press; 2008.
26. Mojtabai R, Olfson M. National trends in psychotherapy by office-based psychiatrists. Arch Gen Psychiatry. 2008;65(8):962–70.
27. Mojtabai R, Olfson M. Proportion of antidepressants prescribed without a psychiatric diagnosis is growing. Heal Aff. 2011;30(8):1434.
28. Healy D. The antidepressant era. Cambridge, MA: Harvard University Press; 1997.
29. Moncrieff J. Are antidepressants overrated? A review of methodological problems in antidepressant trials. J Nerv Ment Dis. 2001;189(5):288.
30. Horwitz A, Wakefield J. The loss of sadness: how psychiatry transformed normal sorrow into depressive disorder. New York: Oxford University Press; 2007.
31. Grob G. Psychiatry's holy grail: the search for the mechanisms of mental diseases. Bull Hist Med. 1998;72(2):189–219.
32. Kraemer HC, Shrout PE, Rubio-Stipec M. Developing the diagnostic and statistical manual V: what will "statistical" mean in DSM-V? Soc Psychiatry Psychiatr Epidemiol. 2007;42: 259–67.
33. Olfson M, Marcus SC, Druss B, Pincus HA. National trends in the use of outpatient psychotherapy. Am J Psychiatry. 2002;159:1914–20.
34. Lopez M, Compton W, Grant B, Breiling J. Dimensional approaches in diagnostic classification: a critical appraisal. Int J Methods Psychiatr Res. 2007;16(1):S6–7.

35. Strakowski S. Do we need a DSM-5? Society for Biological Psychiatry Newsletter. Oct 2011. http://archive.constantcontact.com/fs080/1102694216886/archive/1107066936608.html.
36. Frances A. Whither DSM–V? Br J Psychiatry. 2009;195(5):391–2.
37. Frances A. Rating scales: DSM5 bites off far more than it can chew. In: Psychiatric times [internet]. http://www.psychiatrictimes.com/dsm-5/content/article/10168/1565517. Accessed 7 May 2010a.
38. Schatzberg AF, Scully Jr JH, Kupfer DJ, Regier DA. Setting the record straight: a response to Frances commentary on DSM-V. Psychiatr Times. 2009;26(8):1–3.
39. Costello J. Resignation letter to Daniel Pine. http://www.scribd.com/doc/17162466/Jane-Costello-Resignation-Letter-from-DSMV-Task-Force-to-Danny-Pine-March-27-2009. Accessed 27 March 2009.
40. Livesley WJ. Confusion and incoherence in the classification of personality disorder: commentary on the preliminary proposals for DSM-5. Psychol Inj Law. 2010;3(4):304–13.
41. Phillips K, First M, Pincus H, ed. Advancing DSM: dilemmas in psychiatric diagnosis. Arlington: American Psychiatric; 2003.
42. Frances A. DSM in philosophyland: curiouser and curiouser. Bull Assoc Adv Philos Psychiatry. 2010;17(1):21–5.
43. First MB. Clinical utility: a prerequisite for the adoption of a dimensional approach in DSM. J Abnorm Psychol. 2005;114(4):560–4.
44. British Psychological Society. Response to the American Psychiatric Association: DSM-5 development. June 2011. https://docs.google.com/viewer?url=http%3A%2F%2Fapps.bps.org.uk%2F_publicationfiles%2Fconsultation-responses%2FDSM-5%25202011%2520-%2520BPS%2520response.pdf
45. Society for Humanistic Psychology, Division of American Psychological Association. Open letter to DSM-5; 4 Nov 2011.
46. American Counseling Association. Letter to the American Psychiatric Association; 8 Nov 2011.
47. Brown P. Diagnostic conflict and contradiction in psychiatry. J Health Soc Behav. 1987; 28:37–50.
48. American Psychiatric Association. Diagnostic and statistical manual of mental disorders: DSM-IV-TR. Washington, DC: American Psychiatric; 2000.

Part III
Conceptual Perspectives

Chapter 7
DSM in Philosophyland: Curiouser and Curiouser[*]

Allen Frances

The Epistemologic Game

> First Umpire: *"There are balls and there are strikes and I call them as they are."*
> Second Umpire: *"There are balls and there are strikes and I call them as I see them."*
> Third Umpire: *"There are no balls and there are no strikes until I call them."*

As I recall it, the three umpires are replaying a marathon epistemological game that (1) began with Plato, (2) continued in the medieval joust between the realists and Occam's nominalists, (3) was revived in the post-renaissance debate between Descartes and Vico on the power and limits of rational thought, (4) was refined by Kant, (5) churned up by Freud, and (6) finally settled by quantum physicists who have sharply downgraded the capacity of the human mind to ever fully intuit (much less understand) reality. Closer to my turf, I like to think of Bob Spitzer as umpire #1, me as umpire #2, and Tom Szasz as umpire #3.

Spitzer achieved a paradigmatic revolution in psychiatric diagnosis and nosology. He introduced the method of diagnostic criteria (originally developed for research purposes) into a tool for general clinical practice. For the first time, psychiatrists could agree on diagnoses and make interpretive judgments across the research/clinical interface. Certainly, the level of reliability achieved by DSM-III was oversold, especially when it was used by the average clinician. But DSM-III was a huge leap forward from the useless and neglected guidance offered by DSM-I

[*]An early version of this chapter appeared in the Bulletin for the Advancement of Philosophy and Psychiatry, Vol 10, #1, 2010.

A. Frances, MD (✉)
Department of Psychiatry, Duke University, Durham, NC, USA
e-mail: allenfrances@vzw.blackberry.net

and DSM-II. It gave hope that psychiatry could become scientific and join in the advances that were being made in the rest of medicine.

DSM-III resulted from and promoted the victory of biological psychiatry over the psychological and social models that until then were its serious competitors. In the early dawn of its triumph, the biological model was presented with a realist, reductionist flourish that would have done umpire #1 proud. Mental disorders were real entities that existed "out there." The process of scientific discovery would elucidate their etiology and pathogenesis using the powerful new methods of neuroscience, imaging, and genetics.

The next section will focus on the disappointing fate of this ambitious program, but one central point belongs here. Biological psychiatry has failed to produce quick, convincing explanations for any of the mental disorders. This is because it has been unable to circumvent the fundamental and inherent flaw in the biological, "realist" approach—mental disorders don't really live "out there" waiting to be explained. They are constructs we have made up—and often not very compelling ones at that. It has, for example, become clear that there is no one prototype "schizophrenia" waiting to be explained with one incisive and sweeping biological model. There is no gene, or small subset of genes, for "schizophrenia." As Bleuler intuited, "schizophrenia" is rather a group of disorders, or perhaps better a mob. There may eventually turn out to be 20 or 50 or 200 kinds of "schizophrenia." As it stands now the definition and boundaries of "schizophrenia" are necessarily arbitrary. There is no clear right way to diagnose this gang and not even much agreement on what the validators should be and how they should be applied. The first umpire was called out on strikes when the holy grail of finding the cause of "schizophrenia" turned out to be a wild goose chase.

Szasz is the third umpire. He quickly saw through the epistemological "no clothes" of umpire #1 and led the fight against simple minded biological reductionism (even well before the biologists had discovered their own voice and began making their overly ambitious and naïve claims). Szasz vigorously presented the view that mental illness is a medical "myth." Mental disorders were no more than social constructs that in some cases served a useful purpose, but in many others could be misused to exert a noxious social control, reducing freedom and personal responsibility. The biological "realists" reacted predictably to Szasz' "nominalist" attack. They dismissed it. "If schizophrenia is a myth, they crowed, it is a myth that responds to medication and has a genetic pattern." But their triumphalism was premature and based on both weak philosophic and weak scientific grounds. It turned out that the neuroscience, genetics, and treatment response of "schizophrenia" follow anything but a simple reductionist pattern. The more we learn about "schizophrenia" the more it resembles a heuristic, the less it resembles a disease.

This brings us to me (a call'um as I see'um) second umpire. In preparing DSM-IV, I had no grand illusions either of seeing reality straight on or of reconstructing it whole cloth from my own pet theories. I just wanted to get the job done—i.e., produce a useful document that would make the fewest possible mistakes, and create the fewest problems for patients. Following Vico, I accepted that much in real life (and almost everything in psychiatric classification) is overlapping, fuzzy, and heterogeneous—anything but Cartesian and amenable to overarching rationalist principles or mathematical precision. Psychiatric classification is necessarily a sloppy business. The desirable goal of having a classification consisting of mutually exhaustive, nonoverlapping mental disorders is simply impossible to meet.

Instead, the second umpire follows a down-to-earth brand of Bentham utilitarian pragmatism. His umpire's eye is fixed on the end result of getting to what works best—not distracted by biological reductionism or rationalist models of how things should be constructed. A diagnosis is a call to action with huge and unpredictable results. No decision can be right on narrow scientific grounds if it winds up hurting people.

Descriptive Psychiatry Gets Long of Tooth

> *The Dodo: "Everyone has run and everyone has won and all must have prizes."*

Modern descriptive psychiatry just passed its 200 birthday—if we measure it from the milestone of Pinel's creation of the first psychiatric classification that resembles our own. His work was born from the Enlightenment belief in a rational world—some underlying order could be imposed even on the obvious irrationality of mental illness. The premise was that any domain receiving systematic observation and classification would eventually display causal patterns.

This approach was enormously successful in each of the major paradigm shifts in science. Always a careful description preceded a causal model. Kepler's astronomical observations led to Newton's gravity. Linnaeus' classification of plants and animals led to Darwin's evolution. Mendeleyev's periodic table led to Bohr's structure of the atom. There have been dozens of descriptive systems vying to describe things so brilliantly that their truth would shine forth. "All have run, but none has won prizes." Descriptive classification in psychiatry has so far been singularly unsuccessful in promoting a breakthrough discovery of the causes of mental disorder.

This is doubly disappointing given the miraculous advances in our understanding of normal brain functioning. The advances in molecular biology, brain imaging, and genetics are spectacular—their impact on understanding psychopathology almost nil. Why the disconnect? The answer lies in a paraphrase of the opening lines of Anna Karenina. All normal brain functioning is normal in more or less the same way, but any given type of pathological functioning can have many different causes.

This is also true for all the complex diseases in medicine. A genetics company using the Icelandic registry had tremendous success in finding gene markers for a dozen diseases, including schizophrenia. It recently went bankrupt because, in each instance, the particular candidate marker explained fewer than 3 % of the cases of the particular disease. There appear to be no common genes even for the common illnesses. Psychopathology is heterogeneous and overlapping not only in its presentation but also in its pathogenesis. There will likely be hundreds of paths to schizophrenia, not one or just a few and perhaps no final common pathway. Where does that leave the descriptive system of psychiatry? Fairly high and dry. Nature has obviously chosen to deprive us of clear joints, ripe for carving. There is little indication of any imminent and sweeping etiological breakthrough. Everything points toward a slow and painstaking retail accumulation of explanatory power. It is not even clear that the DSM categorical approach is the best research tool. The NIMH is embarking on a project to correlate an integrated exploration of neural networks with psychopathology. They chose to study dimensions of behavior (e.g., anxiety, pleasure seeking, executive functioning)—not with the standard psychiatric disorders which are deemed too complex to have any simple relationship with a given neural network. Our DSM categories may not lead the future charge in understanding psychopathology.

Our descriptive classification of disorders is old and tired. It has worked hard for us and continues to have many valuable and irreplaceable functions (which we will discuss in the last section). Fiddling needlessly with the labels will not advance science and may actually do more harm than good in its effect on clinical care.

The Elusive Definition of Mental Disorder

> Humpty Dumpty: "When I choose a word it means just what
> I choose it to mean."

When it comes to defining the term "mental disorder" or figuring out which conditions qualify, we enter Humpty's world of shifting, ambiguous, and idiosyncratic word usages. This is a fundamental weakness of our field. Many crucial problems would be much less problematic if only it were possible to frame an operational definition of mental disorder that really worked.

Nosologists could use it to guide decisions on which aspects of human distress and malfunction should be considered psychiatric—and which should not. Clinicians could use it when deciding whether to diagnose and treat a patient on the border with normality. A meaningful definition would clear up the great confusion in the legal system where matters of great consequence often rest on whether a mental disorder is present or absent.

Alas, I have read dozens of definitions of mental disorder (and helped to write one) and I can't say that any have the slightest value whatever. Historically, conditions have become mental disorders by accretion and practical necessity, not because they met some independent set of operationalized definitional criteria. Indeed, the concept of mental disorder is so amorphous, protean, and heterogeneous that it inherently defies definition. This is a hole at the center of psychiatric classification. And the specific mental disorders certainly constitute a hodge-podge. Some describe short-term states, others lifelong personality. Some reflect inner misery, others bad behavior. Some represent problems rarely or never seen in normals, others are just slight accentuations of the everyday. Some reflect too little control, others too much. Some are quite intrinsic to the individual, others are defined against varying and changing cultural mores and stressors. Some begin in infancy, others in old age. Some affect primarily thought, others emotions, yet others behaviors, others interpersonal relations, and there are complex combinations of all of these. Some seem more biological, others more psychological or social. If there is a common theme it is distress and disability, but these are very imprecise and nonspecific markers on which to hang a definition.

Ironically, the one definition of mental disorder that does have great and abiding practical meaning is never given formal status because it is tautological and potentially highly self-serving. It would go something like "Mental disorder is what clinicians treat and researchers research and educators teach and insurance companies pay for." In effect, this is historically how the individual mental disorders made their way into the system.

The definition of mental disorder has been elastic and follows practice rather than guides it. The greater the number of mental health clinicians, the greater the number of life conditions that work their way into becoming disorders. There were only five disorders listed in the initial census of mental patients in the mid-nineteenth century, now there are close to 300. Society also has a seemingly insatiable capacity (even hunger) to accept and endorse newly defined mental disorders that help to define and explain away its emerging concerns. As a result, psychiatry is subject to recurring diagnostic fads. Were DSM-5 to have its way we would have a wholesale medicalization of everyday incapacity (mild memory loss with aging); distress (grief, mixed anxiety depression); defects in self-control (binge eating); eccentricity (psychotic risk); irresponsibility (hypersexuality); and even criminality (rape, statutory rape).

Remarkably, none of these newly proposes diagnoses even remotely pass the standard loose definition of "what clinician's treat." None of these "mental disorders" has an established treatment with proven efficacy. Each is so early in development as to be no more than "what researchers research"—a concoction of highly specialized research interests.

We must accept that our diagnostic classification is the result of historical accretion and accident without any real underlying system or scientific necessity. The rules for entry have varied over time and have rarely been very rigorous. Our mental disorders are no more than fallible social constructs (but nonetheless useful ones if understood and applied properly).

The Conservative/Innovation Debate or Where Have All the Normals Gone?

> *Alice: "But I don't want to go among mad people"*
> *Cheshire Cat: "Oh, you can't help it, we're all mad here"*

DSM-IV would have been a very different document if I had adopted Humpty Dumpty's confident attitude and used my authority to shape it to my personal taste. Bob Spitzer, who had led the efforts to create DSM-III and DSM-IIIR, is a "splitter" whose preference is to divide the diagnostic pie into small manageable pieces. This enhances reliability, but creates many new diagnoses and artificial comorbidity (as complex syndromes are divided into their component parts). I joke that Spitzer never met a new diagnosis he didn't like.

I am more of a lumper and also very wary of diagnostic fads and the unintended consequences of introducing new diagnoses. Given my druthers, DSM-IV would have had fewer, lumped categories and tighter criteria sets to make it harder to get a diagnosis. Instead, I chose not to impose this view on DSM-IV. We would apply a conservative standard for all changes—equally not add new things or take out old ones unless there was substantial evidence to support the change. Many decisions were thus grand-fathered into DSM-IV that would not have had nearly enough support to meet the new higher evidentiary standard.

I am not a particularly risk averse or conservative person in my everyday life. So why the conservative tilt in setting ground rules for DSM-V?

1. The system had previously been in great flux with the rapid fire appearance within 7 years of DSM-III and DSM-IIIR. It needed a period of stability.
2. The two previous DSMs were the product of an innovative and charismatic figure who single-handedly moved the field by dint of his energy, determination, and grit. Now that his accomplishments were realized, it was time for a less personalized leadership and for the field at large to reclaim responsibility for its diagnostic system.
3. My experience working on DSM-III and DSM-IIIR was that most decisions were fairly arbitrary—with plausible supporting arguments that could have gone either way. Making more arbitrary changes didn't make much sense.
4. The scientific evidence supporting proposed changes was usually meager. Requiring that all changes be based on substantial evidence usually shut up even the most passionate advocates.
5. The literatures are not only thin but also mostly derived from highly specialized research settings that have questionable generalizability to the real world.

One's position on the conservative/innovation continuum is influenced by reactions to the epistemological question raised previously. If you regard the categories in DSM as descriptions of "real entities," you will be eager to change definitions in accord with evidence that they can be better described in a way that captures their real natures. On the other hand, if you believe as I do, that the DSM is necessarily more an exercise in forging a common language than in finding a truth, you need a strong reason to change the syntax. And it turns out that such strong evidence is usually lacking. This is why the reliability and utility goals are so important (and for all the discussion about it, validation is not yet particularly meaningful).

The second divide in the conservative/liberal split relates to how worried one is by real world consequences. As a pragmatist, I was acutely conscious that every change made by DSM-IV could have enormous practical consequences: (1) determining who got medicines that could greatly help or greatly harm, (2) deciding insurance and disability claims, and (3) influencing life and death forensic issues. Those of a more pure research world, innovation orientation would argue for "following the data" and damn the consequences. In my view, data sets that are thin and selective are never sufficient support for changes that can cause considerable mischief. So there are two contrasting attitudes. Mine, the conservative view, is "Do no harm—revise the system with a light and cautious touch only when you are sure of what you are doing after a thorough risk/benefit analysis." The conservative approach assumes that things are there for a reason and are imbricated in a complex set of relations. I have had the painful experience of changing a word or two in a seemingly harmless way and then later learning that we had helped trigger an "epidemic" of false positives (as in Attention Deficit Disorder) or a forensic nightmare (e.g., the misuse of Paraphilia NOS in the extended civil commitment of sexual offenders).

Some have taken the opposite view—that the existing system is so bad that even the aggressively innovative DSM-5 is suggesting far too little change, not too much. I believe this to be a naïve Cartesian rationalist view that neglects the deep roots and far flung branches of the diagnostic system. Most of the suggested DSM-5 changes are such really bad ideas that they do not even represent a meaningful test of the conservative/innovator divide. I believe that most sensible people informed of their risks and benefits would veto them (this leaves out the Work Group members who are otherwise sensible but too attached to their pet suggestions to be objective about their risks).

The new suggestions all share the common problem of greatly expanding the reach of "mental disorders" at the expense of normality. Armies of millions (perhaps tens of millions) of false positive "patients" would receive unnecessary and harmful treatments. I have covered this problem extensively elsewhere and won't repeat the details here. A better, because much tougher, test case of the conservative/innovator debate comes from the DSM-IV introduction of Bipolar II disorder. Here there are strong arguments on both sides and no clear right answer.

We knew that adding Bipolar II would be one of the most consequential changes in DSM-IV but went ahead (despite our conservative bias) because of what seemed to be compelling enough research evidence (descriptive, course, family history, treatment response) that it sorted better with bipolar than with unipolar mood disorders. We recognized the risks that some unipolar patients would be mislabeled and receive unnecessary and potentially harmful, mood stabilizing and antipsychotic medication. But this risk seemed more than counterbalanced by the opposing risk posed by uncovered antidepressants for those whose bipolar tendencies were previously missed by the diagnostic system.

Several facts are incontestable about trends since DSM-IV: (1) with a huge push from the pharmaceutical industry, Bipolar II has become an enormously popular diagnosis, (2) so that the ratio of bipolar to unipolar patients increased dramatically, (3) and prescriptions jumped for mood stabilizers and antipsychotics (which can cause huge and dangerous weight gains), and (4) for different reasons rates of childhood Bipolar Disorder have increased 40-fold. Some patients are undoubtedly better off for being diagnosed as Bipolar II. Others have gained a lot of weight (and risk diabetes and a potentially shortened lifespan) taking a medication that was unnecessary.

A conservative might prefer that such public health experiments be based on more evidence than was available to us when we made the decision to include Bipolar II. We also had no way of anticipating how aggressive and successful were the pharmaceutical industry marketing efforts to move product. Bipolar II also illustrates the exquisite and dangerous sensitivity of the diagnostic system to small changes. The hugely consequential decision regarding the need for potentially very harmful medication rests on the most fragile and unreliable of distinctions—the decision whether or not a hypomanic episode is present. If the minimum duration of the episode is set at a week (or even longer), people at risk for antidepressant worsening will be missed; if the requirement is 4 days (or even less), many people will receive unnecessary medication. The symptom thresholds for defining a hypomanic episode are similarly arbitrary and subject to wide swings in sensitivity and specificity, based on very minor adjustments. Making this even more complicated are the difficulties distinguishing hypomania from normal mood in someone who is chronically depressed or hypomania from substance-induced mood elevation in someone using drugs.

The point here is that tiny changes in definition can (and often do) result in large, unpredictable (and usually unwarranted) swings in diagnostic and treatment habits, especially when amplified by drug companies, advocacy groups, and the media. Such potentially dangerous fads are enough to turn a lifelong, risk-taking liberal like me into a conservative nosologist. First, last, and always—do no harm.

Afterword

> The Talmud: "We don't see things as they are, We see things as we are."

Many people are troubled by the relativism implied in this penetrating insight—but I find it liberating. We will never have the perfect diagnostic system. Our classification of mental disorders will always necessarily be no more than a collection of fallible and limited constructs that seek but never find an elusive truth. But this is our best current way of seeing and communicating about mental disorders. And despite all its epistemological, scientific, and even clinical failings, the DSM does its job reasonably well if it is applied properly and its limitations are understood.

The concern about comorbidity across disorders arises from the misconception that each is a "real" and independent psychiatric illness and that clear boundaries should or could be created to separate them. If instead, one accepts that each disorder is just a description (not a disease), then the combined descriptions become modular building blocks each of which adds precision and information.

The concerns about heterogeneity within diagnoses also reflect a longing for well-defined psychiatric "illnesses." Instead, we are dealing with descriptive prototypes ("schizophrenia," "panic disorder," "mood disorder," etc., through the manual) that are inherently heterogeneous and will hopefully with time be divided into many true etiologically defined illnesses.

The greatest misuse of the DSM occurs in diagnosing conditions at the border of normality and criminality. Clinicians should hold themselves to the most rigorous standards when applying criteria sets in these dangerous boundary territories. The DSM incorporates a great deal of practical knowledge in a convenient and useful format.

To not know it casts one outside the community of common language speakers—the language being clinical psychiatry. But it should always be used with pragmatism and clinical common sense.

Chapter 8
Overdiagnosis, Underdiagnosis, Synthesis: A Dialectic for Psychiatry and the DSM

Joseph M. Pierre

Introduction

Like most things in nature, medical illness can be conceputalized on a continuum—one in which "health" and "sickness" are positioned at either end, with many points of relative health and sickness in between. However, practical decision making, whether clinical or otherwise, favors the use of categorical distinctions to define pathology such that the diagnosis of disease is typically based on a threshold preponderance of clinical signs and symptoms, histopathologic features, or laboratory values. "Drawing a line in the sand" to demarcate an illness threshold is therefore a necessary but fluid process that can be subjective, relativistic, and highly context-driven. As a result, the criteria to define even "hard" medical conditions such as hypertension, diabetes, or cancer have shifted over time based upon new morbidity data, innovations in diagnostic technology, and the availability of interventions along different stages of disease.

Defining the borders of illness in psychiatry can be particularly challenging given that mental disorders lack biologic validity (their underlying pathophysiologies are largely unknown), diagnosis is based almost exclusively on cataloging symptomatic criteria (as opposed to biopsy results or laboratory tests), and morbidity is defined by psychological distress or impaired psychosocial functioning (which are more value-laden features than say, imminent risk of death). This doesn't mean that psychiatric disorders don't exist or that diagnostic thresholds are completely arbitrary, as critics sometimes claim, but it does indicate that psychiatric diagnosis can involve considerable subjectivity, just as it often does in other branches of

J.M. Pierre (✉)
Department of Psychiatry and Biobehavioral Sciences,
David Geffen School of Medicine at UCLA, Los Angeles, CA, USA

VA Greater Los Angeles Healthcare System, Los Angeles, CA, USA
e-mail: Joseph.Pierre2@va.gov

J. Paris and J. Phillips (eds.), *Making the DSM-5: Concepts and Controversies*,
DOI 10.1007/978-1-4614-6504-1_8, © Springer Science+Business Media New York 2013

medicine [1], and that debates about the proper positioning of diagnostic thresholds on a health-illness continuum are inevitable.

The debate over diagnostic thresholds in psychiatry has been recently reignited with the pending publication of the 5th Edition of the Diagnostic and Statistical Manual of Mental Disorders (DSM-5), with highly publicized critiques focused largely on claims and concerns about diagnostic overreach [2–4]. Since the publication of DSM-III, whose formal diagnostic criteria greatly improved diagnostic agreement or "inter-rater reliability," subsequent DSM revisions have aimed to improve both validity (the establishment of psychiatric disorders as "disease entities") [5] and "clinical utility" (the usefulness of a diagnosis in clinical practice) [6]. While maximizing reliability, validity, and utility are worthwhile goals in theory, the pursuit of these goals is not without conflict in practice. For example, existing categorical diagnoses may be clinically useful, but not necessarily biologically valid such that using them in research can hinder etiologic discovery [7]. In addition, while recent attempts to improve validity have increasingly recognized a continuum of mental illness, such a "dimensional" view can be at odds with clinical utility and risks undue widening of the scope of mental illness [8]. Finally, clinical practice is but one arena that relies upon DSM diagnosis, such that some disputes about what should or should not be considered a mental disorder arise from competing utilities within clinical and para-clinical contexts [8, 9]. These collective challenges complicate DSM's forward progress and provide ongoing fuel for the debate about the proper diagnostic borders of mental illness.

The Problem of Overdiagnosis: Minimizing False Positives

At their core, many of the recent critiques of DSM-5 involve claims of over-diagnosis—that psychiatry has been ever-widening its borders with diagnostic labels for mental states and responses to life situations that have been and should be considered within normal variation (such overdiagnosis has been synonymously called "diagnostic expansion," "diagnostic creep," "prevalence inflation," "over-pathologizing," "medicalization," "disease mongering," or a problem of "false positives" and "false epidemics") [2–4, 8–11]. For example, it is often noted that the number of cataloged mental disorders in the DSM has more than tripled, expanding from 106 disorders in DSM-I to 357 in DSM-IV [10]. Indeed, recent epidemiologic data indicate that about half of Americans will meet criteria for a DSM-IV disorder sometime in their lives [12], with a 12-month prevalence of 26 % [13]. Some have even asserted that such figures are underestimates due to problems with retrospective detection [14], suggesting that soon it may become normal to have a mental illness at some point in one's life. To what extent this seems wrong-headed depends on one's definition of normal [15], but it nonetheless highlights a longstanding dynamic tension between what has been considered sickness and health in the history of the DSM and American psychiatry.

Initial efforts to form an American classification system for mental disorders arose from attempts to gather census data from public hospitals in the United States in the early 1900s [16]. Since psychiatry at the time centered almost exclusively on asylum care of severe mental illness, such endeavors began with sharp demarcations between mental disorders and mental health [17], where the majority of psychiatric diagnoses consisted of subtypes of psychosis [16]. In contrast, over the next century, American psychiatry transitioned away from a focus on severe mental illness and instead embraced a "neurosis-psychosis continuum" in which "everyone, patients or not, sick or healthy, fell on that continuum somewhere" [18]. In 1963, Karl Menninger described the scope of psychiatry as follows: "Gone forever is the notion that the mentally ill person is an exception. It is now accepted that most people have some degree of mental illness at some time, and many of them have a degree of mental illness most of the time" [19].

American psychiatry's transformation away from psychotic asylum patients towards increasingly less severely ill outpatients occurred in response to three synergistic forces. First, the rise of psychoanalysis drove psychiatrists into private practice-based outpatient therapy where the typical analysand was a college-educated, upper-middle class professional who paid for service out of pocket [20]. Freud himself conceded that "the optimum conditions for (psychoanalysis) exist where it is not needed—i.e., among the healthy" [21]. Second, Adolph Meyer, the "father of American psychiatry," advocated for a patient-centered, psychosocial approach that viewed mental illness on a continuum and advanced far-reaching goals of social reform within the Mental Hygiene Movement, including the belief that mental illness was rooted in personality and stemmed from psychological "reactions" and "maladjustments" to childhood conflicts and other life stressors [22]. Premorbid interventions were therefore directed "beyond the walls of hospitals" [23] into the community and within schools [24], widening the scope of mental health interventions in the United States and paving the way for deinstitutionalization, the development of community-based psychiatry, and the eventual formation of modern federal mental health policy [17]. Finally, recognition of "battle fatigue," "combat exhaustion," and "shell-shock" among soldiers from World Wars I and II crystallized the notion that mental illness was often precipitated by reactions to trauma, particularly among individuals with some latent "predisposition to maladjustment" [24]. Psychiatrists participated in mass screenings of prospective draftees in World War II, with 1.75 million men ultimately rejected from service based upon increasing recognition of "neurotic" as opposed to "psychotic" symptoms and disorders [21]. These "psychoneurotic" syndromes were not cataloged within preexisting psychiatric classification manuals, necessitating revised nosologies encompassing a much broader scope of mental disorder that culminated in the publication of the first Diagnostic and Statistical Manual of Mental Disorders (DSM) in 1952 [25].

To no small extent then, the first editions of DSM were attempts to codify the various syndromes that were being treated during psychiatry's heyday of outpatient psychotherapy. By DSM-III however, the tide threatened to turn, with all but complete eradication of popular analytic and psychosocial theories from its pages in favor of a criterion-based medical model operating on the underlying principle that psychiatric disorders could and would be validated like other medical disorders by the establishment of a clinical description, distinction from other disorders, and laboratory, family/genetic, and longitudinal studies [5]. Along with this sea change departure from psychoanalytic theory, the DSM-III Task Force on Nomenclature and Statistics cast a skeptical eye towards neurotic disorders and originally planned to set a higher threshold for psychiatric diagnosis that would minimize "false positives" [26]. In the end however, such ambitions were scrapped in favor of a "principle of inclusiveness" that sought to incorporate diagnoses already widely in use by clinicians and to maximize the likelihood of their coverage by insurance providers [21, 27]. This approach has remained a guiding principle in subsequent DSM revisions, such that the current DSM-IV contains within its pages the most broadly inclusive array of mental disorders to date.

Claims of overdiagnosis have been ongoing well before and since the DSM-IV era, with recent concerns highlighting the particular overinclusiveness of certain disorders such as major depression [28], bipolar disorder in adults [29–31] and children [32], posttraumatic stress disorder (PTSD) [33, 34], social phobia [35, 36], attention deficit hyperactivity disorder (ADHD) [37], autism [38], sexual dysfunction [39], and the paraphilias [40]. With the coming of DSM-5, renewed concerns that DSM's ever-increasing diagnostic expansion now threatens to run amok have erupted in response to the proposed inclusion of potentially subthreshold conditions including "psychosis risk syndrome," "mild cognitive impairment," "mixed anxiety depression," and "temper dysregulation disorder," as well as proposals to widen the spectrum of addictive disorders to include "behavioral addictions" (e.g., pathological gambling, internet addiction) or to create a broad category of "autistic spectrum disorders" [41]. Critics worry that this potential broadening of the scope of psychiatry risks elevation of false positives and "false epidemics" to unacceptable heights [2, 3]

Concerns about overdiagnosis include both conceptual and consequential elements. The conceptual element involves the argument that the borders of pathology should be distinct and highlights the potential for psychiatry to overstep its bounds by applying a label of mental illness to variants of normal human existence and behavior. Wakefield in particular has advanced the idea that "normal responses to stressful circumstances" and "problems of living" can and should be reliably distinguished from mental illness by equating mental disorder with "harmful dysfunction," defined as some negatively valued outcome caused by a failure of some internal mechanism to perform one of the functions for which it is biologically designed through natural selection [42, 43]. Proponents of the harmful dysfunction argument hold that normal, expected, or proportionate responses to stressors are not mental disorders unless they involve such intensity as to imply the failure of the intended function of a psychological process. According to this view, a number of DSM diagnoses including major depression, adjustment disorder, PTSD, social phobia, and conduct disorder are routinely misapplied to normal responses to life stressors [21, 28, 33, 42, 43]. One author has captured the essence of this conceptual problem of overdiagnosis by noting that "Virtually all of our measures of 'psychopathology' are built on the assumption that to be psychologically healthy is to be free of disordered emotional and cognitive responses. According to this standard, a coma victim might be considered the ideal of psychological health" [44].

In addition to conceptual problems, there are at least two significant consequential concerns about overdiagnosis. First, the more that psychiatric diagnoses appear to encroach on the boundaries of normal behavior, the more psychiatry opens itself to criticisms that there is no validity to the concept of mental disorders (e.g., there's no such thing as mental illness—it's a "myth") [45] or that diagnosis is arbitrary (e.g., psychiatrists "cannot distinguish the sane from the insane") [46]. Similar claims about lack of diagnostic reliability, voiced years ago by the so-called "anti-psychiatry movement" and supported by well-publicized studies [46–48], comprised a major threat to psychiatry that prompted the development of criterion-based diagnoses in DSM-III. Although reliability has been much improved as a result, psychiatry's credibility as a profession remains threatened by the lack of diagnostic validity and the potential to pathologize and stigmatize normal human experience by further diagnostic expansion in DSM-5.

Perhaps the greatest consequential concern of DSM-5 critics is that psychiatric medications will be increasingly marketed to and prescribed for those at the healthier end of the mental illness continuum. For example, valid questions have already been raised about indiscriminant antidepressant use including their increasing prescription for non-disorders [49], their lack of efficacy relative to placebo among those with milder depression [50–52], unnecessary exposure to potentially harmful side effects, and the pharmaceutical industry's vested interest in marketing psychiatric medications to an ever-expanding consumer population [11]. Such questions have been extended to a wide range of existing psychiatric disorders including bipolar disorder, ADHD, and social phobia as well as to more recently proposed disorders for DSM-5 including attenuated psychosis syndrome, disruptive mood dysregulation disorder, and lowered diagnostic thresholds for ADHD and generalized anxiety disorder [3]. We already live in a society in which substances such as caffeine and alcohol are used routinely to "self-medicate" minor suffering associated with daily living, such that if diagnostic expansion in psychiatry continues along its historical trajectory, the lines between therapeutic and cosmetic intervention would likely become increasingly blurred, warranting cautious deliberation about the ethics of "neuroenhancement" [53–56]. It is naïve to think that such considerations apply only to some imagined dystopian future of psychiatry. On the contrary, diagnostic expansion, the availability of cosmetic enhancements, and a consumer-driven market to enhance function and maximize happiness are very much issues with which to contend in the present day.

The Problem of Underdiagnosis: Minimizing False Negatives

While concerns about overdiagnosis center upon the potential risks of labeling and treating "false positives," concerns about underdiagnosis stem from the potential risks of failing to identify and treat "false negatives." This perspective mirrors the principle of inclusiveness that strives to incorporate the wide scope of individuals seeking help from mental health clinicians within the pages of the DSM. With such a clinical focus, diagnosing and relieving suffering is given precedence over academic or semantic debates about what is or is not a mental disorder. If, for example, someone presents with dysphoria related to some life event, a clinician typically will commence intervention rather than fretting over whether this represents a "harmful dysfunction" or an expected response to a stressor, just as an orthopedist would with a patient's broken bone.

Those arguing in favor of maximizing diagnostic inclusiveness recognize the peril of underdiagnosing and not treating "clinically significant" conditions that are associated with distress and functional impairment. Taking the example of major depression, consensus opinion has been published that cites "overwhelming evidence that individuals with depression are being seriously undertreated" [57]. Undertreatment resulting from underdiagnosis appears to be a particular problem in primary care settings where the majority of individuals with depression go to seek help. As many as 65 % of those with major depression go undetected in primary care [58]. Undetected depression is associated with considerable functional impairment including significant rates of "serious" suicidal ideation and for most patients, symptoms remain persistent at 1 year [59]. Underdiagnosis of depression therefore appears to be a serious public health concern even for those seeking medical help and is further compounded by the significant population of those with depression that don't seek medical care at all [60, 61].

Concerns about underdiagnosis have also been extended to the potential neglect of those with mental disorders that lie at the milder end of a severity spectrum as well as those with subthreshold conditions. While subthreshold disorders are by definition less severe than their threshold counterparts, they are nonetheless often associated with significant disability and psychological distress and have the potential to progress to more serious disorders [62–64]. Likewise, those with mental disorders of mild severity still have significantly greater rates of hospitalization, work disability, and a history of serious mental illness compared to those with no mental disorder at all [65]. Given that the prevalence of subthreshold and mild disorders is much larger than disorders of greater severity [63, 66], neglecting the milder end of a mental illness continuum would therefore risk neglect of a substantial proportion of the population with considerable suffering and functional impairment.

The case for erring on the side of diagnostic inclusivity in psychiatry can also be argued from the perspective of reducing stigma—both for patients and for psychiatry as a profession. Stigma associated with mental illness represents a significant barrier to psychiatric care access as well as a source of discrimination and directly harmful health effects mediated by distress [67]. Including only the most severe mental disorders in DSM could perpetuate such stigma by reinforcing the popular notion that seeking psychiatric help is equivalent to being "crazy." In contrast, ensuring that mild and subthreshold conditions are listed in DSM could help to literally normalize mental illness by communicating to the public that mental disorders are common and need not be associated with the inability to lead a meaningful life [68]. Although some ongoing anti-stigma public health efforts are directed at severe mental illness such as schizophrenia [69], expanding such efforts to a wider scope of mental disorders could convey a destigmatizing message that mental illnesses are simply, to paraphrase Susanna Kaysen, "you or me… amplified" [70].

Synthesis

Numbers and Normality

Although those concerned about overdiagnosis in psychiatry decry the proliferation of DSM disorders, the mere fact that there are more disorders listed in DSM-IV than DSM-I doesn't necessarily mean that psychiatry is relentlessly encroaching upon normality. To some extent, the increase in the number of different psychiatric disorders simply reflects attempts to make finer distinctions between disorders that would have fallen under a single diagnosis in previous DSM editions (i.e., "splitting" as opposed to "lumping"). For example, earlier versions of DSM made no distinction between Alzheimer's disease and vascular dementia, whereas now there are separate diagnoses that have both etiologic and clinical pertinence. Similarly, the controversial new DSM-5 diagnosis, disruptive mood dysregulation disorder, has been proposed in part as a way to reduce the overdiagnosis of bipolar disorder in children with recurrent temper outbursts. In this way, a new diagnosis can represent a more appropriate and specific diagnostic label for a condition that might otherwise have ended up in a "wastebasket" category, including any of the numerous "not otherwise specified" disorders within each of the major diagnostic categories in DSM.

The creation of new diagnostic labels does not therefore in itself mean that the number of people diagnosed with mental illness is increasing and does not prove that psychiatry is guilty of encroaching on normality. In order to do that, the actual incidence of mental disorders must be examined along with what we mean by "normality." Returning to the example of depression, critics of overdiagnosis contend that we are currently experiencing a "pandemic" of major depression in which psychiatry has medicalized or pathologized "normal sadness" [28]. However, two large-scale epidemiologic studies specifically examining rates of major depression across different time periods in which DSM-criteria have changed yielded no evidence that the incidence (e.g., new cases) has increased to any significant degree [71, 72]. One study found an increase in prevalence among middle-aged women, but this was attributed to the chronicity of depression rather than the emergence of new cases [72].

Still, the previously cited figures indicating that half if not more of the entire United States population will meet criteria for any lifetime DSM-IV disorder [12, 14] do represent a 10–20 % increase in prevalence compared to studies performed in the DSM-III era [73] and raise important questions about how psychiatry defines mental disorder given that it is becoming normal to have one. The most common explanation for such alarmingly high rates of mental disorder is that mild disorders as well as "transient homeostatic responses to internal or external stimuli that do not represent true psychopathologic disorders" [74]—that is, false positives that reflect normal life suffering—have been inappropriately counted in epidemiologic surveys. However, in the absence of a gold standard to determine what is or is not a disorder, the concept of a false positive in psychiatry is problematic [75]. DSM disorders are clinical syndromes where diagnosis is based upon symptom criteria and in most cases, a requirement of "clinically significant distress or impairment in social, occupational, or other important areas of functioning." "Clinical significance" therefore often serves as the key threshold determinant to distinguish between disorder and normality, but deciding what is significant is a highly subjective and value-laden judgment call [7, 76, 77]. Within epidemiologic surveys performed in nonclinical settings by lay interviewers, clinical significance may be prone to significant overestimation [78]. Indeed, when clinical significance is more carefully assessed and tied to help-seeking behavior, the rates of detected mental disorders in community surveys is reduced by nearly half [66]. A similar effect has been demonstrated in surveys of "voice-hearing," in which surprisingly high rates of auditory hallucinations in community samples were substantially lower following more in-depth interviews by psychiatrists determining clinical significance [79]. Such findings suggest that false positives stemming from faulty judgments about clinical significance may indeed be a problem with epidemiologic surveys, though not necessarily with clinician's use of DSM per se.

In practice, the inherent subjectivity of the clinical significance criterion allows a clinician to make value judgments that can either reduce false positives or maximize inclusiveness, as is convenient to a particular clinical task. Although Wakefield's "harmful dysfunction" definition attempts to minimize false positives by removing this subjectivity from psychiatric diagnosis, it is not clear that such an approach would be either practically feasible or desirable from a clinical perspective [9]. The work of clinicians will always tend to favor a low threshold for defining "caseness" in order to maximize opportunities to relieve the suffering of help-seeking individuals. In contrast, quibbles about exact diagnoses, judgments of severity, or whether it might be normal to have a mental disorder or to seek psychiatric care are of relatively low concern.

Contextual Utility

Although clinical utility has been heralded as a guiding principle to determine what is or is not a mental disorder in the DSM [6], the reality is that different settings both within and outside the clinical arena will inevitably demand different thresholds to define mental illness. Whether a condition should be considered a mental disorder therefore depends on why the question is being asked. As noted, clinicians considering whether an individual should be treated will tend to have a very low threshold to define caseness. The principle of inclusiveness that has focused on minimizing false negatives at the possible expense of including false positives is therefore defensible on the grounds that DSM's "highest priority has been to provide a helpful guide to clinical practice" [6].

However, the DSM is used in myriad para-clinical and nonclinical contexts, such that debates about what should appear in its pages are often confounded by competing "contextual utilities" [8, 9]. For example, funding for psychiatric research typically requires investigation within a specific DSM disorder. However, given the lack of validity among existing disorders, research must be conducted beyond the confines of DSM disorders if psychiatry is to ever make progress in establishing its disorders as disease entities [7, 8]. In this sense, DSM cannot satisfy both clinical and research objectives, such that different criteria to identify conditions may be necessary in each setting. Here, it makes most sense to maintain the DSM as a "good enough guide for clinical work" [7], whereas efforts such as the Research Domain Criteria (RDoC) [80] may prove more useful in the research world. In order to preserve its clinical utility, the DSM should not be used as a tool to maximize research funding [81]. Just so, those conditions initially proposed for inclusion in DSM-5 that have now been relegated to "Section III" (conditions recommended for further study and research) should perhaps be omitted from DSM-5 altogether.

Note also that the principle of inclusiveness can best be argued in private practice settings where financial resources to pay for care are abundant. In other sectors where resources for psychiatric treatment are limited and must be rationed—such as within private insurance providers, public health care, and government disability programs—higher thresholds to define caseness become a necessity [82]. Such economic realities have led to efforts to stratify disorders according to severity by defining "serious mental illness" or to incorporate functional disability (rather than only distress or help-seeking) into public health definitions of mental disorder [82–84]. Therefore, for healthcare administrators responsible for rationing resources, the clinical significance that determines caseness for clinicians cannot be extended to determine treatment need or disability [84–86].

Finally, a variety of forensic situations look to the DSM for definitions of mental disorder, with the potential for significant conflict. This is best illustrated by the indefinite placement of those with paraphilias into psychiatric institutions upon completion of their prison sentences, despite the fact that no clearly effective treatments for such behaviors exist [87, 88]. Indeed, a reasonable argument has been made that paraphilias ought not be considered psychiatric disorders and should be removed from DSM altogether [40, 89]. As with other contextual utilities, the thresholds to define caseness in the clinical realm cannot simply be transferred to questions about involuntary treatment, issues of capacity and competency, and criminal sentencing in the forensic world. These are altogether different questions requiring different answers about mental illness thresholds.

It is therefore impossible for DSM to satisfy all competing contextual utilities that require different thresholds to define psychiatric disorder. Although contextual utilities should be considered, ultimately the DSM should serve as a clinical tool such that decisions about what disorders should be listed in its pages should be made primarily on the pragmatics of clinical utility.

Pragmatism and Consequentialism

In the absence of established validity and pathophysiologies for mental disorders, differentiating between true mental disorders and normal homestatic reactions must ultimately rest upon pragmatic considerations regarding clinical utility [90, 91].

Clinical utility has been defined as "the extent to which DSM assists clinical decision makers in fulfilling the various clinical functions of a psychiatric classification system" that include communication, selecting effective interventions, and predicting future clinical management needs [6]. Deciding what ends up in DSM therefore requires a certain amount of prognostication about possible, but ultimately unknown, effects of any new diagnostic additions.

As noted earlier, the key imagined consequences that fuel concerns about potential overdiagnosis in DSM-5 are twofold. First, following proposals for DSM-5 disorders that seemingly widen the spectrum of mental illness (e.g., psychosis risk syndrome, mixed anxiety depressive disorder, mild cognitive disorder, temper dysregulation disorder, behavioral addictions, autistic spectrum disorders), there are fears that the incidence and prevalence of mental illness will expand to such degree that an overwhelming majority of the population will become mentally ill. DSM-5 architects have recently refuted this, noting that "for the first time in the history of DSM, the total number of diagnoses will not grow" and that "charges that DSM-5 will lower diagnostic thresholds and lead to a higher prevalence of mental disorders are patently wrong. Results from our field trials, secondary data analyses, and other studies indicate that there will be essentially no change in the overall rates of disorders once DSM-5 is in use" [92]. Here, only time will tell, but if there is no increase, it may be because several of the proposed disorders (e.g., psychosis risk syndrome/attenuated psychosis syndrome and mixed anxiety depressive disorder) have been scrapped in response to voiced criticism and concern. Just as likely however is the possibility that there might be no net change in prevalence because those diagnosed with the new DSM-5 disorders would have previously been diagnosed with some other disorder, such as a "not otherwise specified" condition.

With regard to the issue of pharmacotherapy, concern about the overuse of psychotropic medications is indeed warranted in light of the potential for DSM-5 to increase medication prescription for a wider spectrum of psychiatric disorders. Progressive movement towards neuroenhancement will continue to be driven by society's sense that happiness is an entitlement [93], the increasing acceptance of pharmacotherapy to assuage "day to day stresses" and interpersonal problems [94], and the motives of those who stand to benefit from diagnostic expansion including both pharmaceutical companies and the industry of psychiatry as a whole [8, 9, 11]. Ultimately, whether psychiatric medications should be prescribed for disorders along the milder end of a mental illness continuum must depend upon rigorous analysis of risk-benefit. Lowering the threshold to define mental illness is likely to occur along with the assumption that pharmacotherapy would be a benefit for both mild and severe disorders, though recent evidence with antidepressants highlights that this would be a grave mistake [50–52]. More efficacy studies for milder conditions are clearly needed to accurately gauge the potential benefits of pharmacotherapy. At the same time, risk analysis must include not only consideration about exposure to side effects, but also the ethics and imagined consequences of neuroenhancement to both individuals and society [53–56]. To date, such consideration of neuroethics for DSM-5 has been conspicuously lacking [8, 77, 95].

Maximizing Pragmatism for DSM-5: Psychosis Risk Syndrome

The debate about whether "prodromal psychosis," "psychosis risk syndrome (PRS)," or more recently, "attenuated psychosis syndrome" should be included in DSM-5 illustrates how the tension between the potential for overdiagnosis and underdiagnosis can be balanced through an analysis of consequentialism, pragmatism, and competing contextual utilities. For the past 15 years, well-intentioned research efforts have sought to identify individuals at highest risk to develop a psychotic disorder (usually based on the presence of transient or attenuated positive symptoms) and to develop effective early interventions for adolescents and young adults at risk [96, 97]. Individuals recruited into prodromal psychosis research clinics tend to be already symptomatic, functionally impaired, and either help-seeking or in distress, suggesting the presence of clinical significance and the need for intervention [98]. Most patients meet criteria for a mood or anxiety disorder [99] that doesn't account for their attenuated positive symptoms (often resulting in a referring diagnosis of psychotic disorder not otherwise specified), such that a more specific and appropriate diagnosis could help with communication, prognostic estimation, and treatment planning. Therefore, proponents of incorporating PRS into DSM-5 believe that inclusion is warranted based on satisfactory clinical utility [100].

The main argument against inclusion of PRS centers on the problem of false positives. Indeed, "conversion rates" (the proportion of identified high-risk subjects who go on the develop full blown psychosis) in published studies have been declining and currently average 22 % at 1 year and 36 % after 3 years [101], with false-positive rates (subjects who do not progress to psychosis) in some studies as high as 95 % at 6-months [102] and 92 % at 2-year follow-up [99]. These rates suggest that the majority of patients who are identified at high-risk may not develop psychosis, with as many as 59 % of subjects in one study no longer even meeting high-risk criteria after 1 year [103]. In fact, the most common outcome for those deemed at high-risk for psychosis isn't psychosis, but rather the continuation of mixed anxiety and depressive symptoms [104]. This could be attributed in part to the effectiveness of ongoing interventions that are integrated into research clinic care, but it is also "likely that this high false-positive rate is due largely to the inherent difficulty in distinguishing between attenuated positive symptoms and the normal range of thoughts, speech, and behavior characteristic of adolescents and young adults transitioning through a challenging phase of life" [105]. These are sobering considerations that call into question the clinical utility of PRS, particularly when juxtaposed with the potential for stigmatization due to being diagnosed as at high-risk for psychosis [106].

Concerns have also been raised about the potential for unnecessary exposure to antipsychotic medications in this population for which optimal treatment guidelines are lacking [3, 100, 101]. Such concerns can be applied to either side of the DSM-5 debate however. On the one hand, if PRS were to appear in DSM-5 as a temporal (e.g., as a potential premorbid prodrome) and symptomatic expansion (i.e., as a syndrome characterized mainly by subthreshold psychotic symptoms) of the psychosis spectrum, there are legitimate fears that rampant prescription of antipsychotic medications for young people might follow. While these medications may have a role in the treatment of PRS, efficacy data have been inconsistent [103, 107, 108] and antipsychotic prescription could occur at the expense of other interventions that might be at least as effective, but substantially safer including antidepressants [109], omega-3 fatty acids [110], and psychotherapy [111]. On the other hand, a substantial proportion of individuals in prodromal psychosis clinics are already prescribed anti-psychotics by their referring clinicians [112], such that the inclusion of PRS in DSM-5 could reduce inappropriate prescribing and instead facilitate the develop-ment, implementation, and awareness of evidence-based guidelines that could improve clinical care [100].

These arguments reveal the complexity of judging clinical utility and highlight other contextual utilities of diagnosis beyond the realm of clinical care. For exam-ple, Carpenter (the chair of the DSM-5 Psychoses Workgroup) has argued in favor of including PRS in DSM-5 based on retaining a "framework for early detection and intervention" and upon scientific validity "even if concern for potential misuse is serious"[113]. Other investigators have advocated for DSM-5 inclusion as a means to promote future PRS research [100]. As previously noted however, DSM-5 should maintain its primary role as a rough guide for clinical work and DSM inclusion should not occur in the service of supporting research efforts. Furthermore, at this stage of PRS research, the main goal is to get better at identifying individuals at risk by determining genetic, psychophysiologic, endophenotypic, and neuroimaging predictive markers with much lower false-positive rates compared to existing crite-ria based upon subthreshold symptoms. Until that has been achieved, keeping the research criteria for PRS that have already been developed, standardized, and imple-mented within prodromal psychosis clinics out of DSM-5 should not impede further research where the "framework" that Carpenter speaks of is already in place. Given the high rate of false positives, the possibility that PRS represents a risk of generic psychiatric impairment rather than one specific to psychotic disorders [104], and the lack of coherent treatment guidelines, a pragmatic risk-benefit analysis does not therefore favor DSM-5 inclusion. Indeed, such analysis has been reflected in the recent decision to change the name of PRS and to place "attenutated psychosis syn-drome" into DSM-5's Section III (conditions recommended for further study and research).

Future Direction

The basic conflict between overdiagnosis and underdiagnosis is rooted in the rela-tive merits and risks of maximizing the scope of psychiatry and minimizing false negatives on the one hand and restricting the scope of mental illness and minimizing false positives on the other. Even if DSM were to focus its primary goal on clinical utility as it should, debate about the proper thresholds to define mental illness will persist so long as multiple conflicting questions are being asked of diagnostic thresholds. The key question for the future—perhaps for DSM-6—is whether there is a way to resolve this confusion. Finding a solution will require that psychiatry choose a clearer mission not only for the DSM, but for itself as a profession within the larger scope of mental health care.

The current direction of DSM-5 suggests that psychiatry aims to increasingly adopt a "dimensional" view of a mental health-mental illness continuum that recognizes the ubiquity of suffering associated within both normal life and mental disorder with the hope of maximizing opportunities for intervention [8, 9, 114]. According to this vision reminiscent of the Mental Hygiene Movement, the scope of mental health care in the future could target not only disorders, but also isolated symptoms, complaints, normal responses to stressful life situations, and expected existential suffering. Likewise, interventions themselves would be expanded beyond targeted treatment of suffering to include preventive care as well as the promotion of well-being and healthy lifestyles. Although critics of overdiagnosis oppose such expansion, there need not be anything philosophically or ethically wrong with this approach, nor even with the consequence that a majority of the population ends up seeking and receiving mental health care. Over the course of our lives, having a transient or chronic physical illness and receiving medical treatment is completely normal and to be expected. Since its inception, general medical practice has managed suffering associated with pain, coughs, broken bones, pregnancy, aging, and the process of dying independent of debate about whether these conditions represent "harmful dysfunctions." There is no a priori reason why that should differ for psychiatry.

Several authors have noted that "prior to the mid-twentieth century, most moderate mental disorders received no treatment other than the care people received from their general physician and from family, friends, and clergy" [86] or that while "nowadays patients with mental disorders seek help from a psychiatrist... in former times, such patients would have tried to cope with their problem alone" [63]. Others have admonished that "it would be unfortunate for psychiatry to prematurely roam into problems usually better handled by family and other cultural institutions" [115] and "a reduced tolerance of individuals and society for suffering, abnormality, and impairment lowers the threshold for complaining and self-seeking" [63]. While this kind of "pick oneself up by one's own bootstraps" approach to suffering sounds admirable, it may just as likely represent a significant barrier to mental health treatment intertwined with lack of access to care and fear of stigmatization [116]. Mental health care therefore has the potential to fill important gaps that have been left by an increasingly secularized, decentralized, and less family-oriented society. Psychiatry's adoption of a mental health-mental illness continuum model might also go a long way towards reducing stigma associated with psychiatric disorders.

At the same time, if the DSM seeks to capture any condition along the mental health-mental illness continuum associated with suffering, then the conditions within its pages cannot be realistically equated with those conditions requiring treatment by a psychiatrist with subspecialty medical training that is both expensive and typically focused on pharmacotherapy. There simply aren't enough psychiatrists to meet the needs of the full continuum, nor would any such public healthcare system be able to afford the high cost of care if there were. From a treatment standpoint, great care must be taken to not assume that effective treatments at one end of the continuum should be applied in blanket fashion at other points. It is likely that many milder conditions might very well be best managed with psychotherapeutic approaches that support self-efficacy, coping, and the ability to weather suffering. While pharmacotherapy for mild conditions should not be prohibited on merely philosophical grounds, well-designed comparative research studies with careful analyses of risk-benefit and discussions about the ethics of neuroenhancement will be required to establish evidence-based optimal care guidelines. It is likely that a full spectrum of mental health care needs will be best addressed in a graded or staged fashion with a wide range of interventions that include preventative measures, no treatment/watchful waiting, self-help/coping/resiliency-promoting strategies, exercise and other lifestyle interventions, psychotherapy, and pharmacotherapy [9, 62, 65, 117, 118]. Accordingly, cost-effective implementation of such a broad palette of interventions will require the integration of an array of providers including not only psychiatrists, but also primary care clinicians, psychotherapists, paraprofessionals, laypersons, peers, and patients themselves.

In the final analysis, the determination of proper diagnostic boundaries in psychiatry is complicated by reliance on clinical signs and symptoms, competing contextual utilities that depend upon the DSM, and lack of consensus about the very definition of a mental disorder [77, 119, 120]. Adopting a continuous model of mental health-mental disorder for psychiatry could help to disarm debates about thresholds by acknowledging that subthreshold conditions and non-disorders may be worthy of intervention without having to claim that everyone has a mental disorder. Such a continuous view is likely more consistent with underlying reality, especially in terms of particular symptoms (e.g., anxiety, reality testing, impulsivity, memory impairment). Acknowledging the fluidity of diagnostic thresholds within a continuum and according to context needn't mean that mental disorders don't exist at all, but rather that, to use a medical analogy, there is a continuum of routine coughs reflecting no disorder per se, transient coughs associated with self-limited irritation or infection, nagging coughs indicative of bronchitis, and hemoptysis arising from pneumonia or malignancy—each requiring different levels of intervention.

The DSM seems to now be at crossroads where it is poised to free psychiatry from the fetters of categorical diagnoses and illness thresholds in favor of increased attention to a wider mental health-mental illness continuum. Clinical utility and the principle of inclusiveness remain primary goals, but to what clinicians does this refer? Few critics of overdiagnosis rigidly oppose intervention for an individual who's feeling down after ending a romantic relationship, but they do question what kind of intervention is best and doubt that optimal intervention always warrants a physician psychiatrist and a prescription for psychotropic medication. Expanding DSM's concept of mental disorder within a continuum model makes sense within the larger scope of public mental health care, but economic realities, risk-benefit analyzes, and neuroethical concerns should limit parallel expansion of the scope of treatment by psychiatrists in kind. In this sense, DSM can sidestep the threshold problem by embracing a more continuous model of mental health-mental illness, but outside of the microcosm of private practice, debates about the proper thresholds to trigger specific intervention by psychiatrists will linger on.

References

1. Pies R. How "objective" are psychiatric diagnoses? (guess again). Psychiatry. 2007;4: 18–22.
2. Frances A. A warning sign on the road to DSM-5: beware of unintended consequences. Psychiatric Times [Internet]. 26 Jun 2009 [cited 1 Aug 2012]. www.psychiatrictimes.com/display/article/10168/1425378.
3. Frances A. Opening Pandora's box: the 19 worst suggestions for DSM5. Psychiatric Times [Internet]. 11 Feb 2010 [cited 1 Aug 2012]. http://www.psychiatrictimes.com/dsm/content/article/10168/1522341.
4. Angell M. The illusions of psychiatry. New York Review of Books [Internet]. 14 Jul 2011 [cited 1 Aug 2012]. http://www.nybooks.com/articles/archives/2011/jul/14/illusions-of-psychiatry Accessed 1 July 2012.
5. Robins E, Guze SB. Establishment of diagnostic validity in psychiatric illness: its application to schizophrenia. Am J Psychiatry. 1970;126:983–7.
6. First MB, Pincus HA, Levine JB, Williams JBW, Ustun B, Peele R. Clinical utility as a criterion for revising psychiatric diagnoses. Am J Psychiatry. 2004;161:946–54.
7. Pierre JM. Deconstructing schizophrenia for DSM-5: challenges for clinical and research agendas. Clin Schizophr Relat Psychoses. 2008;2:166–74.
8. Pierre JM. The borders of mental illness in psychiatry and the DSM: past, present, and future. J Psychiatr Pract. 2010;16:375–86.
9. Pierre JM. Mental illness and mental health: is the glass half empty or half full? Can J Psychiatry. 2012;57(11):651–8.
10. Double D. The limits of psychiatry. BMJ. 2002;324:900–4.
11. Moynihan R, Heath I, Henry D. Selling sickness: the pharmaceutical industry and disease mongering. BMJ. 2002;324:886–91.
12. Kessler RC, Berglund P, Demler O, et al. Lifetime prevalence and age-of-onset distributions of DSM-IV disorders in the National Comorbidity Survey replication. Arch Gen Psychiatry. 2005;62:593–602.
13. Kessler RC, Chiu WT, Demler O, et al. Prevalence, severity, and comorbidity of 12-month DSM-IV disorders in the National Comorbidity Survey replication. Arch Gen Psychiatry. 2005;62:617–27.
14. Moffitt TE, Caspie A, Taylor A, et al. How common are common mental disorders? Evidence that lifetime prevalence rates are doubled by prospective versus retrospective ascertainment. Psychol Med. 2010;40:899–909.
15. Smith R. In search of "non-disease". BMJ. 2002;324:883–5.
16. Grob GN. Origins of DSM-I: a study in appearance and reality. Am J Psychiatry. 1991;148:421–31.
17. Grob GN. The forging of mental health policy in America: World War II to new frontier. J Hist Med Allied Sci. 1987;42:410–46.
18. Ghaemi SN. Nosologomania: DSM & Karl Jaspers' critique of Kraepelin. Philos Ethics Humanit Med. 2009;4:10.
19. Menninger K. The vital balance: the life process in mental health and illness. New York: Viking; 1963.
20. Shorter E. A history of psychiatry: from the era of the asylum to the age of Prozac. New York: Wiley; 1997.

21. Horwitz A. Creating mental illness. Chicago: The University of Chicago Press; 2002.
22. Double DB. What would Adolf Meyer have thought of the neo-Kraepelinian approach? Psychiatr Bull. 1990;14:472–4.
23. Meyer A. The mental hygiene movement. Can Med Assoc J. 1918;8:632–4.
24. Cohen S. The mental hygiene movement, the development of personality and the school: the medicalization of American education. Hist Educ Q. 1983;23:123–49.
25. The Committee on Nomenclature and Statistics of the American Psychiatric Association. Diagnostic and statistical manual: mental disorders. Washington, DC: American Psychiatric Association; 1952.
26. Wilson M. DSM-III and the transformation of American psychiatry: a history. Am J Psychiatry. 1993;150:399–410.
27. Spitzer RL, Williams JBW. American psychiatry's transformation following the publication of DSM-III. Am J Psychiatry. 1994;151(3):459–60.
28. Horwitz AV, Wakefield JC. The loss of sadness: how psychiatry transformed normal sorrow into depressive disorder. Oxford: Oxford University Press; 2007.
29. Zimmerman M, Ruggero CJ, Chelminski I, Young D. Is bipolar disorder overdiagnosed? J Clin Psychiatry. 2008;69(6):935–40.
30. Patten SB. Does almost everyone suffer from a bipolar disorder? Can J Psychiatry. 2006; 51:6–8.
31. Patten SB, Paris J. The bipolar spectrum—a bridge too far? Can J Psychiatry. 2008; 53:762–8.
32. Duffy A. Does bipolar disorder exist in children? A selected review. Can J Psychiatry. 2009; 52:409–17.
33. Spitzer RL, First MB, Wakefield JC. Saving PTSD from itself in DSM-5. J Anxiety Disord. 2007;21:233–41.
34. Rosen GM, Taylor S. Pseudo-PTSD. J Anxiety Disord. 2007;21:201–10.
35. Wakefield JC, Horwitz AV, Schmitz MF. Are we overpathologizing the socially anxious? Social phobia from a harmful dysfunction perspective. Can J Psychiatry. 2005;50:317–9.
36. Lane C. Shyness: how normal behavior became a sickness. New Haven: Yale University Press; 2007.
37. Sciutto MJ, Eisenberg M. Evaluating the evidence for and against the overdiagnosis of ADHD. J Atten Disord. 2007;11:106–13.
38. King M, Bearman P. Diagnostic change and the increased prevalence of autism. Int J Epidemiol. 2009;38:1224–34.
39. Balon R. The DSM, criteria for sexual dysfunction: need for a change. J Sex Marital Ther. 2008;34:186–7.
40. Moser C, Kleinplatz PJ. DSM-IV-TR and the paraphilias: an argument for removal. J Psychol Human Sex. 2005;17:91–109.
41. Miller G, Holden C. Proposed revisions to psychiatry's canon unveiled. Science. 2010; 327:770–1.
42. Wakefield JC. Diagnosing DSM-IV—Part 1: DSM-IV and the concept of disorder. Behav Res Ther. 1997;35(7):633–49.
43. Wakefield JC. The concept of mental disorder: diagnostic implications of the harmful dysfunction analysis. World Psychiatry. 2007;6:149–56.
44. Hayes SC, Strosahl KD, Wilson KG. Acceptance and commitment therapy: an experiential approach to behavioral change. New York: The Guilford Press; 1999.
45. Szasz TS. The myth of mental illness: foundations of a theory of personal conduct, revised edition. New York: Harper and Row; 1974.
46. Rosenhan DL. On being sane in insane places. Science. 1973;179:250–8.
47. Kendell RE, Cooper JE, Gourlay AJ, Copeland JR, Sharpe L, Gurland BJ. Diagnostic criteria of American and British psychiatrists. Arch Gen Psychiatry. 1971;25:123–30.
48. Kendell RE. Psychiatric diagnosis in Britain and the United States. Br J Psychiatry. 1975;9:453–61.

49. Pagura J, Katz LY, Mojtabai R, Druss BG, Cox B, Sareen J. Antidepressant use in the absence of common mental disorders in the general population. J Clin Psychiatry. 2011; 72(4):494–501.

50. Khan A, Leventhal RM, Khan SR, Brown WA. Severity of depression and response to anti-depressants and placebo: an analysis of the food and drug administration database. J Clin Psychopharmacol. 2002;22(1):40–5.

51. Kirsch I, Deacon BJ, Huedo-Medina TB, Scoboria A, Moore TJ, Johnson BT. Initial severity and antidepressant benefits: a meta-analysis of data submitted to the Food and Drug Administration. PLoS Med. 2008;5(2):e45.

52. Fournier JC, DeRubeis RJ, Hollon SD, Dimidjian S, Amsterdam JD, Shelton RC, et al. Antidepressant drug effects and depression severity: a patient-level metaanalysis. JAMA. 2010;303(1):46–53.

53. Kass LR. Beyond therapy: biotechnology and the pursuit of happiness. http://biotech.law.lsu.edu/research/pbc/reports/beyondtherapy/beyond_therapy_final_report_pcbe.pdf. Accessed 1 July 2012.

54. Farah MJ, Illes J, Cook-Deegan R, Gardner H, Kandel E, King P, et al. Neurocognitive enhancement: what can we do and what should we do? Nature Rev. 2004;5:421–5.

55. Greely H, Sahakian B, Harris J, Kessler RC, Gazzaniga M, Campbell P, et al. Towards responsible use of cognitive-enhancing drugs by the healthy. Nature. 2008;456:702–5.

56. Larriviere D, Williams MA, Rizzo M, et al. Responding to requests from adult patients for neuroenhancements: Guidance of the Ethics, Law and Humanities Committee. Neurology. 2009;73:1406–12.

57. Hirschfield RMA, Keller MB, Panico S, Arons BS, Barlow D, Davidoff F, et al. The National Depressive and Manic-Depressive Association consensus statement on the undertreatment of depression. JAMA. 1997;277(4):333–40.

58. Coyne JC, Schwenk TL, Fechner-Bates S. Nondetection of depression by primary care physi-cians reconsidered. Gen Hosp Psychiatry. 1995;17:3–12.

59. Rost K, Zhang M, Fortney J, Smith J, Coyne J, Smith GR. Persistently poor outcomes of undetected major depression in primary care. Gen Hosp Psychiatry. 1998;20:12–20.

60. Angermeyer MC, Matschinger H, Riedel-Heller SG. Whom to ask for help in case of a men-tal disorder? Preferences of the lay public. Soc Psychiatry Psychiatr Epidemiol. 1999;34(4): 202–10.

61. Aoun S, Pennebaker D, Wood C. Assessing population need for mental health care: a review of approaches and predictors. Ment Health Serv Res. 2004;6(10):33–46.

62. Magruder KM, Calderone GE. Public health consequences of different thresholds for the diagnosis of mental disorders. Compr Psychiatry. 2000;41(2 Suppl 1):14–8.

63. Helmchen H, Linden M. Subthreshold disorders in psychiatry: clinical reality, methodologic artifact, and the double-threshold problem. Compr Psychiatry. 2000;41(2 Suppl 1):1–7.

64. Rucci P, Gherardi S, Tansella M, Piccinelli M, Berardi D, Bisoffi G, et al. Subthreshold psy-chiatric disorders in primary care: prevalence and associated characteristics. J Affect Dis. 2003;76:171–81.

65. Kessler RC, Merikangas KR, Berglund P, Eaton WM, Koretz DS, Walters EE. Mild disorders should not be eliminated from the DSM-V. Arch Gen Psychiatry. 2003;60:1117–22.

66. Narrow WE, Rae DS, Robins LN, Regier DA. Revised prevalence estimates of mental disor-ders in the United States: using a clinical significance criterion to reconcile 2 survey's esti-mates. Arch Gen Psychiatry. 2002;59:115–23.

67. Schulze B. Stigma and mental health professionals: a review of the evidence on an intricate relationship. Int Rev Psychiatry. 2007;19(20):137–55.

68. Henderson C, Thornicroft G. Stigma and discrimination in mental illness: time to change. Lancet. 2009;373:1928–30.

69. Sartorius N. Stigma: what can psychiatrists do about it? Lancet. 1998;352:1058–9.

70. Kaysen S. Girl, interrupted. New York: Turtle Bay Books; 1993.

71. Mattisson C, Bogren M, Nettelbladt P, Munk-Jorgensen P, Bhugra D. First incidence depression in the Lundby Study: a comparison of the two time periods 1947-1972 and 1972-1997. J Affect Disord. 2005;87:151–60.
72. Eaton WW, Kalaydjian A, Scharfstein DO, Mezuk B, Ding Y. Prevalence and incidence of depressive disorder: the Baltimore ECA follow-up, 1981–2004.
73. Robins LN, Helzer JE, Weismann MM, Orvaschel H, Gruenberg E, Burke Jr JD, et al. Lifetime prevalence of specific psychiatric disorders in three sites. Arch Gen Psychiatry. 1984;41:949–58.
74. Regier DA, Kaelber CT, Rae DS, Farmer ME, Knauper B, Kessler RC, et al. Limitations of diagnostic criteria and assessment instruments for mental disorders: implications for research and policy. Arch Gen Psychiatry. 1998;55:109–55.
75. Pies R. The ideal and the real: how does psychiatry escape the DSM-5 "Fly-bottle?". Bull Assoc Adv Philos Psychiatry. 2010;17(2):18–22.
76. Spitzer RL, Wakefield JC. DSM-IV diagnostic criteria for clinical significance: does it help solve the false positives problem? Am J Psychiatry. 1999;156:1856–64.
77. Pierre JM. Mental disorder vs. normality: defining the indefinable. Bull Assoc Adv Philos Psychiatry. 2010;17(20):9–11.
78. Frances A. Problems in defining clinical significance in epidemiologic studies. Arch Gen Psychiatry. 1998;55:119.
79. van Os J, Hanssen M, Bijl RV, Ravelli A. Strauss (1969) revisited: a psychosis continuum in the general population? Schizophr Res. 2000;45:11–20.
80. Insel T, Cuthbert B, Garvey M, et al. Research Domain Criteria (RDoC): toward a new classification framework for research on mental disorders. Am J Psychiatry. 2010;167:748–50.
81. Pincus HA, Frances A, Davis WW, First MB, Widiger TA. DSM-IV and new diagnostic categories: holding the line on proliferation. Am J Psychiatry. 1992;149:112–7.
82. Goldman HH, Grob GN. Defining "mental illness" in mental health policy. Heal Aff. 2006;25(3):737–49.
83. Substance Abuse and Mental Health Services Administration. Final notice establishing definitions for (1) children with a serious emotional disturbance, and (2) adults with a serious mental illness. Fed Regist. 1993;58:29422–5.
84. Ustun B, Kennedy C. What is "functional impairment"? Disentangling disability from clinical significance. World Psychiatry. 2009;8:82–5.
85. Spitzer RL. Diagnosis and need for treatment are not the same. Arch Gen Psychiatry. 1998;55:120.
86. Mechanic D. Is the prevalence of mental disorders a good measure of the need for services? Heal Aff. 2003;22(5):8–20.
87. First M, Halon R. Use of DSM paraphilia diagnoses in sexually violent predator commitment cases. J Am Acad Psychiatry Law. 2008;36:443–54.
88. First M, Frances A. Issues of DSM-IV: unintended consequences of small changes: the case of paraphilias. Am J Psychiatry. 2008;165:1240–1.
89. Green R. Is pedophilia a mental disorder? Arch Sexual Behav. 2002;31:467–71.
90. Maj M. Are we able to differentiate between true mental disorders and homestatic reactions to adverse life events? Psychother Psychsom. 2007;76:257–9.
91. Philips J, Frances A, Cerullo M, Chardavoyne J, First M, Ghaemi N, et al. The six most essential questions in psychiatric diagnosis: a pluralogue part 2: issues of conservatism and pragmatism in psychiatric diagnosis. Philos Ethics Humanit Med. 2012;7:8.
92. Kupfer DJ, Dr. Kupfer defends DSM-5. Medscape psychiatry [Internet]. 1 Jun 2012 [cited 1 Aug 2012]. http://www.medscape.com/viewarticle/764735.
93. McMahon DM. Happiness: a history. New York: Atlantic Monthly Press; 2006.
94. Mojtabai R. Americans' attitudes towards psychiatric medications: 1998-2006. Psychiatr Serv. 2009;60:1015–23.
95. Pierre JM. Final comment. Bull Assoc Adv Philos Psychiatry. 2010;17(20):12–3.
96. Addington J, Cadenhead KS, Cannon TD, et al. North American Prodrome Longitudinal Study: a collaborative multisite approach to prodromal schizophrenia research. Schizophr Bull. 2007;33(30):665–72.

97. Correll CU, Hauser M, Auther AM, et al. Research in people with psychosis risk syndrome: a review of the current evidence and future directions. J Child Psychol Psychiatry. 2010;51(40):390–431.
98. Ruhrmann S, Schultze-Lutter F, Klosterkotter J. Probably at-risk, but certainly ill—advocating the introduction of a psychosis spectrum disorder in DSM-V. Schizophr Res. 2010; 120:23–37.
99. Morrison AP, French P, Stewart SLK, Birchwood M, Fowler D, Gumley AI, et al. Early detection and intervention evaluation for people at risk of psychosis: multisite randomized controlled study. BMJ. 2012;344:e2233.
100. Woods SW, Walsh BC, Saksa JR, et al. The case for including attenuated psychotic symptoms syndrome in DSM-5 as a psychosis risk syndrome. Schizophr Res. 2010;123:199–207.
101. Fusar-Poli P, Bonoldi I, Yung AR, Borgwardt S, Kempton MJ, Valmaggia L, et al. Predicting psychosis: meta-analysis of transition outcomes in individuals at high clinical risk. Arch Gen Psychiatry. 2012;69(3):220–9.
102. Yung AR, Phillips LJ, Nelson B, et al. Randomized controlled trial of interventions for young people at ultra high risk for psychosis: 6-month analysis. J Clin Psychiatry. 2011; 72(4):430–40.
103. Simon AE, Umbricht D. High remission rates from an initial ultra-high risk state for psychosis. Schizophr Res. 2010;116:168–72.
104. McGorry PD. Risk syndromes, clinical staging and DSM V: new diagnostic infrastructure for early intervention in psychiatry. Schizophr Res. 2010;120:49–53.
105. Corcoran CM, First MB, Cornblatt B. The psychosis risk syndrome and its proposed inclusion in the DSM-V: a risk-benefit analysis. Schizophr Res. 2010;120:16–22.
106. Yang LH, Wonpat-Borja AJ, Opler MG, et al. Potential stigma associated with inclusion of the psychosis risk syndrome in the DSM-V: an empirical question. Schizophr Res. 2010;120:42–8.
107. McGorry PD, Yung AR, Phillips LJ, Yuen HP, Francey S, Cosgrave EM, et al. Randomized controlled trial of interventions designed to reduce the risk of progression to first-episode psychosis in a clinical sample with subthreshold symptoms. Arch Gen Psychiatry. 2002;59:921–8.
108. McGlashan TH, Zipursky RB, Perkins D, Addington J, Miller T, Woods SW, et al. Randomized, double-blind trial of olanzapine versus placebo in patients prodromally symptomatic for psychosis. Am J Psychiatry. 2006;163:790–9.
109. Cornblatt BA. The New York high risk project to the Hillside recognition and prevention (RAP) program. Am J Med Genet. 2002;114:956–66.
110. Amminger GP, Schäfer MR, Papageorgiou K, et al. Longchain omega-3 fatty acids for indicated prevention of psychotic disorders: a randomized, placebo- controlled trial. Arch Gen Psychiatry. 2010;67:146–54.
111. Morrison AP, French P, Walford L, et al. Cognitive therapy for the prevention of psychosis in people at ultra-high risk: randomized, controlled trial. Br J Psychiatry. 2004;185:291–7.
112. Walker EF, Cornblatt BA, Addington J, et al. The relation of antipsychotic and antidepressant medication with baseline symptoms and symptom progression: a naturalistic study of the North American Prodromal Longitudinal Sample. Schizophr Res. 2009;115:50–7.
113. Carpenter WT. Anticipating DSM-V: should psychosis risk become a diagnostic class? Schizophr Bull. 2009;35:841–3.
114. Helzer JW, Kraemer HC, Krueger RF, Wittchen HU, Sirovatka PJ, Regier DA, editors. Dimensional approaches in diagnostic classification: refining the research agenda for DSM-V. Arlington, VA: American Psychiatric Association; 2007.
115. Frances A. How to avoid medicalizing normal grief in DSM5. Psychiatric Times [Internet]. 16 Mar 2010 [cited 1 Aug 2012]. http://www.psychiatrictimes.com/topics/content/article/10168/1538825.
116. Mojtabai R, Olfson M, Sampson NA, Jin R, Druss B, Wang PPS, et al. Barriers to mental health treatment: results from the National Comorbidity Survey Replication. Psychol Med. 2011;41(8):1751–61.

117. McGorry PD. Issues for DSM-V: clinical staging: a heuristic pathway to valid nosology and safer, more effective treatment in psychiatry. Am J Psychiatry. 2007;164(6):859–60.
118. Batstra L, Frances A. Diagnostic inflation: causes and a suggested cure. J Nerv Ment Dis. 2012;6:474–9.
119. Stein DJ, Philips KS, Bolton D, Fulford KWM, Sadler JZ, Kendler KS. What is a mental/psychiatric disorder? From DSM-IV to DSM-V. Psychol Med. 2010;40:1759–65.
120. First MB, Wakefield JC. Defining 'mental disorder' in DSM-V. Psychol Med. 2010;40:1779–82.

Chapter 9
What Does Phenomenology Contribute to the Debate About DSM-5?

Aaron L. Mishara and Michael A. Schwartz

Learning from History: DSM-III's Research Agenda

DSM-III's (1980) revolutionary neo-Kraepelinians were dedicated to setting up a research program rather than accurately reflecting clinical realities. Embracing Carl Hempel's [1] logical empiricist agenda, they approached mental disorders in terms of operational definitions for the purpose of enhancing reliability in diagnosis [2]. "Spitzer selected a group of psychiatrists and consultant psychologists who were committed primarily to medically oriented, diagnostic research and not to clinical practice" [3]. That is, *there was and remains a divide between DSM-III and later DSMs' prescriptive diagnostic practices for researchers and what clinicians actually do in practice*. Far from bridging clinical practice and clinical research, DSM-III inserted a wedge between them. "Operational definitions are too restrictive. They preclude extensions to new situations that are even slightly different from the original defining condition" [4]. The original criteria used as the initial basis for the specified diagnostic criteria for the major diagnostic categories of DSM-III were regarded exclusively as "research diagnostic criteria" (RDCs) [5]. Even Gerald Klerman, "the highest-ranking psychiatrist in the federal government at the time," who had at first appraised the movement from the DSM-I and II to the DSM-III as a "victory for science," later revised his view that DSM-III was largely "a political document" (cited by [3]). That is, by adopting Hempel's logical-empirical approach to science, the neo-Kraepelinians' presumable "revolution" in conceptualizing and classifying

A.L. Mishara (✉)
Department of Clinical Psychology, Sofia University, Palo Alto, CA, USA
e-mail: Aaron.Mishara@sofia.edu

M.A. Schwartz
Departments of Psychiatry and Humanities in Medicine Texas A & M
Health Science Center College of Medicine, Round Rock, TX, USA

J. Paris and J. Phillips (eds.), *Making the DSM-5: Concepts and Controversies*,
DOI 10.1007/978-1-4614-6504-1_9, © Springer Science+Business Media New York 2013

mental disorders actually preempted alternative approaches. In their zeal for reliable diagnosis, DSM-III advocates overlooked that the Hempelian approach they adopted was only one approach that neglected more phenomenologic approaches, also informed by philosophy but in a manner completely different than Hempel. In fact, the German psychiatrist, Karl Jaspers [6, 7], largely responsible for introducing philosophic phenomenology to psychiatry, had written that to the extent that psychiatry ignores philosophy, it is inevitably undone by it in one way or another [8].

Diagnosis Is Not a Checklist But an Interactive, Embodied Social Cognitive Process

Based on Jaspers' phenomenological approach, Schwartz and Wiggins [9] proposed that clinicians use a different method in their practice than that outlined by the neo-Kraepelinian embrace of Hempelian nomological science: the clinician's experience is already pervaded by typifications which help to structure the clinicians diagnosis meaningfully. The founder of philosophic phenomenology, Husserl, had indicated that perceptual meaning is itself based on such a typification process. We never perceive the individual thing or person but always in terms of the type that implicitly subsumes it. We perceive the not yet known in terms of the known, i.e., in terms of the general type that is activated in the particular perception. With each view, there is built a reference to the next anticipated view based on past experience of this and similar objects. The references between aspects are anticipatory constraints, which are nevertheless open to revision or cancelation in their structure so that each aspect prefigures its successor in seamless transition as belonging to the same perceptual object (i.e., subsumed under the particular type that provisionally organizes the perceptual experience until that type is confirmed or refuted by subsequent experience; for review of Husserl's type concept as it applies to the experience of both things and persons, see [10]).

As any other expertise, diagnostic decision making is informed by largely unconscious processes. There is a "gut feeling" which rapidly guides the expert to the most fitting response in completely new contexts or "situations." The philosopher Hans Georg Gadamer [11] calls this process "hermeneutics," the "art" of "interpretative application," *how* the rule is *somehow* optimally applied to the particular case. The well-known neurologist Damasio [12] finds this process to be governed by what he calls "somatic markers." Here, bodily or gut feelings based on past experience subtly "bias" current decision making often in an unnoticed manner. Mishara [13] has further characterized the hermeneutics-somatic marker relationship.

Bransford et al. [14] note that very often the experts themselves are unable to provide an account of the decision processes leading to expert judgment in the particular situation. They cannot articulate the "tacit knowledge" that guides their practice. Developing this sort of expertise takes years of training, a repeated learning by doing in the individual situation, i.e., a learning by examples, which after a while becomes automatic. We see the same sort of learning underlying diagnostic practice [15].

Paradigm Shift: Phenomenological-Clinical Neuroscience

The phenomenologic approach, based on philosophical phenomenology (not to be confused with how the term phenomenology is frequently used in current psychiatric literature) prepares the way for a paradigm shift from the biomedical model of DSM-III, and subsequent DSMs, to a more "person-centered medicine." "Respect for the patient's autonomy, values, and dignity represents a fundamental recognition of his or her personhood, and an ethical imperative. Slowly these concepts are finding their way into evidence" [16].

By checking off symptoms, whether the patient's responses fulfill diagnostic criteria, we stop asking the patient what she or he experiences. We take interest in the client's responses to the extent that they fulfill our predefined operationalized diagnostic criteria. This excludes further exploration of the patient's experience. Therefore the DSMs since 1980 do not do phenomenology of the patient's subjective experience but preclude it.

By relying solely on the DSM, researchers and clinicians actually preempt further research of how the patient's subjective experience can be mapped onto underlying neural processes and the development of more effective interventions. We believe that the proposed paradigm shift to a more phenomenologically based clinical neuroscience in ways that we further describe below provides a more holistic, narrative, strength-based (empowering), contextual, and culturally sensitive approach that generates new hypotheses for clinical research [17].

Although DSM-III and the later DSMs ultimately rely on the patient's reports of their own subjective experience of symptoms and the clinician's observations of signs that the patient may not directly experience, there is little or no effort in DSM to formalize and/or operationalize subjective experience itself. Despite this lack of precise conceptual relationship to what it presumably and ultimately targets (the patient's subjective experience, i.e., suffering in self and/or others), DSM-III and its successors pose the dangers of a "hegemony" [8], a co-opting of clinical practice and clinical research such that research grants, publications, conference presentations, insurance reimbursement, and the like are compelled to make use of reliable DSM diagnoses (despite DSM's own initial caveats that the categories are only provisional and therefore, still lack conceptual foundation).

Toolbox or Pandora's Box: The Elusiveness of Human Subjectivity

Recently, we [18, 19] critiqued the metaphoric toolbox as it applies to diagnosis and classification: "the clinical researcher, Mary Phillips proposes a 'psychiatric toolbox' (i.e., neuropsychological tests, neuroimaging, genotyping) to develop disorder 'biomarkers' that are persistent, rather than state dependent [20]. This would obviate the phenomenological research of the patient's subjective experience of the disorder. The danger will be, however, that we will define disorders in terms of what technologies we have available" [18]. We advise similar caution when using the toolbox metaphor in the application of phenomenology to clinical neuroscience as it applies to the diagnosis and classification of mental disorders.

Rather, phenomenologically based clinical neuroscience must take a different direction more respectful of the entire person in their context [18, 19]:

> The two phenomenological psychiatrists, Klaus Conrad [21] (for review, see [22]) and Henri Ey [23], employed the nineteenth century neurologist, Hughlings Jackson's approach to classification in terms of describing and formalizing the subjective experience of the patient as a field of consciousness which is disrupted in its organizing activity precisely in response to the degree of severity of the underlying neurobiologic disturbance. ... phenomenological psychiatrists begin with healthy waking consciousness and by ... 'removing' healthy components of this consciousness (in as it were introspective, phenomenologic thought experiments, what Husserl called 'imaginative variation'), attempt to produce the subjective experience of symptoms until they arrive at a plausible model. In this way, ... both Conrad and Ey apply a Jacksonian hierarchical approach to nervous functioning in the organization of the patient's 'field of consciousness' [18].

Hughlings Jackson [24] proposed "a two-tiered system for diagnosis—with one tier reserved for clinical practice and a second for research: ... we propose that using the patient's subjective experience of 'symptoms' as standard, there should be ongoing studies of bidirectional feedback between clinical practice and the diagnostic classifications operationalized by researchers to further refine these classifications" [18].

Therefore we propose that "phenomenology is not the antithesis to operationalism but precisely the step required to translate the patient's subjective experience of symptoms, etc., into workable operationalizable hypotheses which can be quantifiably measured using the experimental methods of clinical neuroscience" [19].

Kraepelin, Jaspers, and the DSMs: Does Phenomenology Add Anything?

As Berrios and Hauser observe: "Psychiatry still lives in a Kraepelinian world and its practitioners cannot escape the blinding embrace of its episteme" [25]. What is this epistemological framework we have inherited from Kraepelin? Why do we still live within it? Why is it blinding? And why might this be a problem for current and future DSMs?

With the fifth edition of his textbook (1896), Kraepelin proposed that psychiatric disorders are best conceptualized as "natural disease units" (natürliche Krankenheitseinheiten), that is, discrete entities as in other medical conditions [26]. This approach presumes to "cut nature at the joints" without any evidence that it does so. "Simply put, he [Kraepelin] asserted that psychiatric disorders exist in nature and can be studied in the laboratory" [27]. However, it is not clear that the "ideal types" [7] we use to organize clinical experience necessarily correspond to real clinical entities out there in the world. As Musalek describes the problem:

"Nature itself does not know these forms and categories invented by human beings" [28]. This is particularly evident when considering Kraepelin's dementia praecox (what Bleuler renamed as schizophrenia), which—parallel to the progressive paralysis of neurosyphyillis—is a unitary clinical entity with common insidious course and outcome or end-state [29].

Jablensky [30] writes, "...once a diagnostic concept like schizophrenia has been 'operationalised' for general use, it tends to be reified. ...The mere fact that a diagnostic concept is listed in an official nomenclature and provided with an operational definition tends to encourage this insidious reification". As we mentioned above, by operationalizing diagnosis, the DSMs since DSM-III have actually preempted the phenomenlogical study of the patients' experience of symptoms and how these can be mapped onto neural processes. As we shall see, Jaspers addresses why there is a pervasive tendency to reify diagnostic entities which we nevertheless ascertain in an interactive process.

When Jaspers arrived as a voluntary assistant at the Heidelberg psychiatry clinic in 1908, Kraepelin had just left a couple of years previously to head the Munich university psychiatry clinic. Nevertheless, as Jaspers indicates, the Heidelberg clinic, as German psychiatry generally, was very much working under Kraepelin's influence, whether supporting Kraepelin's work or criticizing it. Still, Kraepelin's concept of dementia praecox was being challenged on several fronts. Kraepelin's previous assistant, Gaupp [31, 32], had proposed that paranoid delusions could be due to character rather than some brain disease as in the well publicized case of the school teacher Wagner who committed mass murder. This was followed by Kretschmer who wrote his habilitation under Gaupp that delusions of reference are due to an overly sensitive but obstinate, ambitious character [7, 33]. Freud [34] had also proposed that paranoid delusions could be "explained" in terms of repressed unconscious contents. For Jaspers, it became critical to distinguish those delusions which were due to character, or reactive to experience, from those involving an underlying, yet to be discovered, neurobiological process. By invoking his often cited opposition between "development of personality" and schizophrenia "process" based on some as yet unknown neurobiological change, Jaspers was able to differentially diagnose delusion-like ideas from primary delusions. The latter are "nonderivable" from any psychological continuity in the patient's personality and thus contribute to a diagnosis of a process schizophrenia. Jaspers writes that his opposition of "development of personality" (ascertained in psychological understanding) vs. process schizophrenia (accessible only through causal explanation) *are not* be thought of in the terms of Kraepelin's "massive" clinical entities. Rather, by introducing these terms, Jaspers underscores the importance of the contextuality and developing expertise of diagnostic practice. In a statement that anticipates his emphasis on ideal types (Weber) in psychological understanding just a couple of years later in the General Psychopathology [6], he (1910) writes: "It is clear that what is meant here (i.e., 'process' and 'development') are provisional heuristic concepts, these concepts do not actually nor exhaustively define the individual case and that between them are many transitions or gradations" [35]. Indeed, Jaspers affirms: "we experience in the other a unity which we cannot define but only experience" [35].

However, he also affirms the value of explanatory, physiological, and neurobiological approaches. Delusions are characterized as being non-understandable in terms of their historical-cultural context and the person's biography, or motivations. It is because the underlying neurobiological process has interrupted the development of the individual person.

What is pertinent for the DSMs, including DSM-5, which will appear in the same year as the centennial for the publication of the first edition of Jaspers "General Psychopathology" [6], is that phenomenology should not be understood as opting for the descriptive over the neurobiological, mind over body, subjective over objective, or the individual personal history over diagnostic classification. Rather the clinician must be able to shift from reductive neurobiological explanation to contextual understanding of the patient's ethnic, cultural, and individual background in order to be able to diagnose delusions in schizophrenia as resulting from some unknown (at that time and still today!) neurobiological process. That is, natural scientific explanation (which is reductive) and understanding (which is holistic and contextual) work in opposite directions [36], yet the clinician must be able to move from one to the other in diagnosing delusions precisely when psychological understanding fails, i.e., when we are no longer able to produce the inner psychological connectedness between the delusion and some prior mental state in the client, whether this be the client's psychological reaction, character, or motivation. Jaspers [6, 7, 35] proposes that diagnosis, as in the case of primary delusions in schizophrenia, must freely move between being explanatory and contextual and therefore anticipates a "person-centered medicine" [37]. However, diagnoses are provisional or "heuristic" in the sense that the classes or entities referred to are not established clinical unities in Kraepelin's sense. In this regard, Jablensky cites Jaspers [7]: "When we design a diagnostic scheme … we abandon the idea of disease entity and once more have to bear in mind continually the various points of view (as to causes, psychological structure, anatomical findings, course of illness and outcome), and in the face of the facts we have to draw a line where none exists … a classification therefore has only a provisional value. It is a fiction which will discharge its function if it proves to be the most apt for the time" [38].

DSM-5's Shift to Clusters and the Neglected Problem of "Reality": Where Is the Phenomenology?

In preparation for DSM-5, Andrews et al. [39] raise the following questions in the proposed shift from Kraepelinian clinical entities to clusters: "Could large clusters of diagnoses be identified by shared external validating factors rather than by symptom pictures alone? Are there now sufficient data from neuroscience, genetics, epidemiology and therapeutics to identify groups of disorders?".

We agree with Hyman that "it is probably premature to bring neurobiology into the formal classification of mental disorders that will form the core of DSM-V…" Still Hyman contends that neurobiology may be used as a "central tool to rethink mental disorders...that could liberate science from the unintended consequences of reifying the current diagnoses that probably do not mirror nature" [40]. However, the neurosciences are themselves subject to the same circular problem that we encounter in the DSMs, that ultimately, we can only study what we have already classified, whether these be discrete clinical entities, dimensions, or clusters—even with the ongoing "bottom-up" discoveries from the neurosciences (see below). We therefore find Andrews and colleagues' claim problematic and circular: "In broad terms, neuroscience, genetics, epidemiology and therapeutics are the variables that validate cluster membership" [30]. Because the neurosciences are developing so rapidly, any cluster which bases itself on current state of the art neuroscience will nevertheless be superseded by the very neuroscience it claims as its basis in a matter of years.

In support of the DSM-5 revisions, Regier and colleagues note that a telltale sign that we are not appropriately carving nature at the joints with the diagnostic taxonomy of DSM-IV-TR is the high incidence of comorbidity. There is "a lack of clear separation between current disorders as defined by DSM IV" and a failure to "identify zones of rarity between mental disorders" [41]. In their celebrated 2003 contribution, Kendell and Jablensky write: "The possibility that disorders might merge into one another with no natural boundary in between—...a 'point of rarity,' but what is better regarded as a zone of rarity—was simply not considered.... Robins and Guze's classic paper was written at a time when it was widely assumed that schizophrenia and manic depressive (bipolar) disorder were transmitted by single— or at the most two or three—genes and before publication of the first studies examining whether there were 'zones of rarity' between related syndromes. The situation now is quite different. ...Most such attempts have ended in failure" [42].

Nevertheless, Jablensky [30] points to weaknesses in DSM-5: "...the methodology underlying the five clusters is not compelling. It is not based on systematic reviews, meta-analyses or statistical taxometric approaches. ...A different panel of efforts might come up with quite different conclusions...At best, they are augmented nomenclatures, that is lists of names of conditions and behaviors supplied with elaborate rules as to how these names should be used. ...their closest analogues are the so-called naturalistic or 'folk' classifications" (pp. 2099–2100). With regard to the schizophrenia, schizotypal, and delusional disorders cluster, Jablensky questions "the a priori selection of 'reality distortion'... as the defining criterion of this cluster" (p. 2102).

In the meantime, Van Os [43] has proposed the term "salience syndrome... to replace all current diagnostic categories of psychotic disorders." This allows for a syndromal system of classification "combining categorical and dimensional representations of psychosis." This would also contribute to reducing the stigma-inducing terminology of the previous DSMs, what Van Os calls "iatrogenic" stigma, in that salience would be viewed along a measurable continuum as a variation of "normal human mentation." Salience is a "natural phenotype" which is dimensional. After all, we presumably all experience salience. Therefore we could imagine what it might be like to have this in excess. "If the values of the dimensional components of the Salience syndrome rise above a certain threshold, need for care may arise" [43].

While we are particularly sympathetic with aberrant salience models of prediction error [44] and presumably resultant "reality" distortion as precisely those models supported by the phenomenology of prodromal delusional mood and psychosis (see [21, 22, 37, 45] and below), we are concerned that fundamental conceptual and practical problems continue to be overlooked and will be perpetuated with the publication of DSM-5. For example, Van Os' [43] proposal to link psychosis to normal mentation presupposes that we first know what "normal" mentation is. It seems that we as clinicians and researchers are so busily looking at and trying to characterize disorders, syndromes, etc., without doing the preparatory work of asking what is the basis of common sense reality as the norm from which putative "reality distortion" or "salience" syndromes deviate, whether these deviations be categorical or dimensional. It seems that DSM-5, as previous DSMs, presupposes normal consciousness as a given, based on common sense, without seeing that any claims about what deviates from "normal" experience in a particular culture, whether these be categorical or dimensional, requires that we first spell out what are the assumptions that support our everyday "healthy" or normative consciousness presumably disrupted in disorders. Our everyday common sense reality is so obvious that we do not bother to ask about the underlying mechanisms, the complex, automatic cognitive-affective processes and "intact" neurocircuitry required to produce such a "reality." We spontaneously commit ourselves to this reality the moment we awake each day without the slightest thought and assume in our everyday experience, folk psychology and attendant ordinary language that the others we encounter more or less share in this reality (see naïve realism below). It is this ordinary everyday understanding of common sense which becomes the basis for the historical-cultural assumption of "normalcy" and its deviations in the DSMs [46, 47].

DSM-5 Presupposes Common Sense Naïve Realism to Describe Deviations from "Normalcy"

Definitions of psychotic experiences as deviations from a "normal" baseline consciousness presumed to more or less "accurately" represent the world, i.e., as "distortions" of our otherwise relatively "accurate" representation of reality are problematic. This would require that we could somehow demonstrate that our everyday default consciousness does in fact have an accurate representation, when in fact most recent evidence in social and cognitive neuroscience demonstrates that our representations of reality are far from accurate.

Philosophic phenomenology [48, 49] offers a means of circumventing this dilemma by proposing a more neutral definition: the altered states of consciousness (ASC) in psychosis involve the suspension, disruption, or bracketing of the "natural attitude," our usual commonsense ways of constructing reality. In the everyday "natural attitude," we assume reality is "obviously" given to us. Recent findings in cognitive science/neuroscience, however, support the view that our everyday experience of a consensual reality is far from accurate and is rather based on a host of human common sense assumptions about accessing a consensual reality [50].

Phenomenological approaches to the study of consciousness as subjectively constituting (i.e., "constructing") its own reality allow for systematic distortions of accuracy in our experience as an adaptive function which keeps the person meaningfully embedded in self-world interactions [36, 51]. That is, perceptual "illusions" [52] and cognitive distortions (cognitive "heuristics") are systematically integrated into our everyday experience of reality as if they were a kind of glue that holds it together. Naïve realism [53], the bias that one's own perspective on reality is objective, resembles what Husserl [54], the phenomenological philosopher, described as the natural attitude, the attitude we naturally assume in our everyday experience. The latter is shaped or informed by "common sense" as our default, everyday approach to experiencing the world. Common sense has a protective function in maintaining an unquestioned, "natural" relationship between internal experience and external "reality." Our mental health is preserved by a certain resistance to losing common sense [55]. The very term common sense comprises a social factor (often supporting the status quo or habitually accepted consensus). As the social psychologist Fiske [56] indicates, individuals tend to endorse meanings that are consensual or held by the group in order to enhance the experience of belonging in that group, and the sense of belonging, even when this sense of belonging depends on excluding individuals who are different from oneself. More recent evidence suggests that oxytocin was selected for early in our evolution not as the love or "cuddle chemical," but as a way of insuring cooperation in tribes who were endangered by ongoing attacks and competition for resources [57]. That is, in-group favoritism and thus a sense of belonging by derogating out-groups may be powerfully rewarded by the neurocircuitry underlying social experience in the human brain.

The organization of self-world relationship (and the preservation of its coherence) is mediated by the dynamic Gestalt meaning of the perception, which is experienced as an ongoing living connectedness between embodied self and environment [10, 51]. The phenomenological philosopher Husserl [54] had demonstrated that our everyday default attitude is a habitual, relatively limited awareness of what comprises the "reality" of this self-world relationship, the naïve realism of the natural attitude.

As Mishara and Fusar-Poli [37] have recently described it: "In everyday experience, we believe that what we directly see and experience is real." Jaspers writes "we live uncritically....in an *immediate* world" [58], a world given to us naïvely and effortlessly [54]. We remain blind to the interpretive lens through which we experience this "immediate" world, the product of implicitly functioning, unnoticed biases. "The other (foreigner) is misunderstood, reduced to the motives and goals of one's own world" [58]. In "common sense" [59], "we often seem to [directly] experience another's feelings, intents or traits...Using an intuitive...relatively automatic process, people do not think about making attributions, they just do it" [56]. We believe our perceptions and judgments, being a direct reflection of reality, are more objective, less biased than others [60]. We experience our own actions as arising in response to a situational-context, but attribute others' behaviors as due to their traits and dispositions, overlooking the situational-contextual factors they experience from their perspective [61]. Our default mode of reasoning about others is biased toward a self-perspective [62]. Jaspers writes: "As matter of course, we take the current moment, what is familiar, the more or less stable social-milieu, and our internal mental life…as the only one that exists. Everything else is naively experienced and judged as fully in harmony with our perspective" [58].

It appears that our everyday reality depends on a host of assumptions which function precisely by being "overlooked" (von Weizsaecker) [58]. This has been confirmed by more recent work in cognitive heuristics, change blindness, and ongoing probalistic models of our experience from moment implicitly based on our past experience, in which expectations and goal processing adjust from moment to moment in terms of prediction error, and past knowledge of self. That is we naturally expect experience to continue more or less the same as it has in the previous few moments and in countless situations prior to the present. Our common sense precisely because it withdraws from too close scrutiny or awareness, i.e., is primarily automatic and habitual, "protects our mental health" (Blankenburg) [55]. Moreover, according to Blankenburg, it is precisely this common sense which is compromised in schizophrenia, making their statements, behaviors, etc., "ununderstandable" in Jaspers sense [7, 8, 37, 55].

To the extent that the DSMs since 1980, including DSM-5, rely on an unquestioned common sense normalcy as anchoring their concept of "reality," they are also subject to the same cognitive distortions that give rise to this reality and all the attendant common sense oppositions that plague the current conceptual foundations of psychiatric diagnosis [47]. We will now examine how these unexamined assumptions give rise to many of the dilemmas confronting current psychiatric classification and diagnosis.

Why the DSMs Do Not Question Their Own Foundation in Common Sense

In their oft-cited contribution, Kendell and Jablensky [32] cite Jaspers' taking exception to the Kraepelinian approach as an alternative. It is not clear why the authors then do not follow through in pursuing what Jaspers' approach (based on Weber's ideal types but also Husserl's phenomenology) [63] would mean for diagnostic classification. Even when Jablensky [64] cites the "ideal types" approach, he collapses it with the more recent "prototype" theory as if the two were synonymous (see [65] for distinction between these approaches).

In contrast to Jaspers' phenomenology, Jablensky often, e.g., [32] cites the Hempelian model: "It is worth recalling that although most sciences start with a categorical classification of their subject matter, they often replace this with dimensions as more accurate measurement becomes possible" (p. 23; see also [64]). Posing the problem similarly to Van Os presupposing common sense normalcy, "we can apply a set of thresholds in order to separate 'pathology' from 'normal variation' and determine the need for treatment" [38].

In perhaps a similar spirit to the Hempelian model, Kendler [66] proposes that taxonomies (biological, psychiatric) naturally proceed from more top-down "approaches advocated by experts and based on a few essential features of the organism chosen a priori" which are ultimately replaced by "bottom-up approaches making use of a much wider array of features." Kendler does not provide details about how such a bottom-up approach would look like as it currently applies to psychiatric diagnosis. However in a subsequent contribution, Kendler and First [67] write: "...a 'bottom-up' empirical methodology for creating categories....could seek to develop a 'theory-free' set of input variables including not only symptoms and signs but also other potential variables such as genetics, biological measures, brain imaging, treatment response and course of illness..." Kendlar and First then opt for a more conservative strategy: "Despite the serious shortcomings of the current descriptive categorical paradigm adopted by DSM–IV and ICD–10, the current evidence suggests that both DSM–V and ICD–11 are likely to continue this approach... As noted by Regier and colleagues, 'the major difference between DSM–IV and DSM–V will be the more prominent use of dimensional measures in DSM–V'" (p. 649).

The overlooked role of common sense assumptions in making decisions about psychiatric diagnostic classification becomes particularly evident when we examine the following contradictory texts. Regier et al. [68] write that the

> ...proposed reclassification of mental disorders for research purposes is predicated on a neuroscience-based framework that can contribute to a nosology in which disorders are grouped by underlying pathophysiological similarities rather than phenomenological observations..... As we gradually build on our knowledge of mental disorders, we begin bridging the gap between what lies behind us (presumed etiologies based on phenomenology) and what we hope lies ahead (identifiable pathophysiologic etiologies).... while also supporting our philosophy that DSM-5 remains first and foremost a tool for clinicians (p. 673).

That is they presume that the work of phenomenology is already done and needs to be superseded presumably by more bottom-up neuroscience approaches.

However, Regier et al. [69] also write in a separate contribution without seeing the contradiction: "we wholly support the ...greater inclusion of mental health consumers and other stakeholders in the DSM-V revision, and we have gone to considerable effort to operationalize our commitment to this effort from the beginning of the DSM-V development process...." Moreover, "Clinical judgment... must include consideration of the patient's unique experience and narrative of their symptoms" (p. 309). Thus, the authors appear not to see a conflict between somehow involving patients in the development of DSM-5, but at the same time excluding phenomenology. That is, the authors give token acknowledgement to patient experience while at the same time dismissing it from having any bearing on bottom-up approaches as simply too unreliable to enter current questions about diagnostic validity. As they have clearly articulated, the phenomenological work is already done. It "lies behind us," whereas we make the case that the phenomenological work in the true sense has never begun because of an inability to appropriately define subjectivity.

In their chapter, "Reflections from within: three stories from within psychosis," Robert Miller, Fred Frese, and Peter Chadwick (all three of whom are accomplished professionals who have been diagnosed with schizophrenia and who have been involved in public advocacy to reduce the stigma of mental illness) write about "...the need for a real contribution from those with lived experience. Yes! We should be at the table with documents like DSM and ICD are assembled, as equal partners" [70].

That is, phenomenology, if it is fine-grained enough, is able to generate specific hypotheses about implicated neural circuits in different neuropsyciatric disorders. For many researchers and practitioners, it probably seems like a tremendous leap from the imprecision of subjective reports of individually experienced symptoms to the specificity of neural circuits. However, part of the problem is that Regier and other architects of the DSMs start with an unexamined concept of subjectivity, one that is shaped in our common sense assumptions about the world. The definition of subjectivity used by the authors is informed by the common sense assumption that subjectivity is simply the inverse of objectivity, i.e., lacking "objectivity" and therefore unreliable is. This exclusively negative definition of subjectivity as private or methodologically inaccessible is the product of the same methodological behaviorism that pervades the past 100 years of trying to make psychology and psychiatry a science based on measurable observables [47].

The common sense view that subjectivity is simply the inverse of the objective, i.e., hidden and unreliable, is coupled with the view that phenomenology is only able to reveal or explore the uniqueness of the individual person in their situation and does not say something about subjectivity in general and how subjective experience is systematically altered in different mental disorders. For example, in his response to our contribution [71], Allen Frances writes, "The phenomenological approach advocated by Drs. Mishara and Schwarz may provide a richer and more nuanced view of the individual, but one that is inherently inferential and unreliable. This is a useful listening style for the clinician trying to understand the patient's inner experience, but it is not a reliable guide to diagnostic decision making. 'Gut feelings' are invaluable in therapists, often misleading for diagnosticians" (p. 7).

This is to articulate our cultural common sense assumption that human subjectivity is individual and unique, something that has depth and can be explored in psychotherapy. Yes, we agree, it is this. Jaspers writes about understanding the individual patient as a whole person in their cultural context and individual life history. But subjectivity is also something much more than the individual subject inside an inviolable black-box which others construe or reconstruct from the outside. The ability to achieve default healthy or normal consciousness requires an attachment to common sense which although distributed differently in different individuals [50], nevertheless has common features and functions across individuals. Similarly we do not know whether there is something like a "higher consciousness," and/or "compassion," which individuals (whether healthy or with mental disorders) report when doing mindfulness-based stress reduction (MBSR) or related practices. What we do find however is that "healers in very diverse communities in the world deliberately induce ASC in themselves and/or their patients," and that the phenomenological properties and implicated neural circuitry appears to be quite similar across ASC [50]. That is, both healthy everyday consciousness and deviations from "normal" consciousness appear to have their own phenomenological structure and implicated neural pathways and mechanisms. The phenomenological approach to psychiatry as represented by Jaspers, Binswanger, Blankenburg, Conrad, Ey, von Weizsäcker, and many others, proposes the research of interacting phenomenological dimensions: space, temporal experience, embodiment, self, and others, which through phenomenological descriptions can be mapped onto brain function.

The failure of the DSMs since 1980, and the research based on their operationalization of mental disorders, to systematically incorporate patient subjectivity and patient collaboration into the clinical research process has prevented psychiatry from taking the next step in mapping neuropsychiatric symptoms onto neural circuitry and neural mechanisms. The fear of subjective experience as being unreliable, and therefore the resistance to think differently (i.e., beyond our culturally inherited common sense biases) about these problems, or to shift paradigms to a more embracing definition of human experience as embodied intersubjective relationship with the various intersecting phenomenological dimensions mentioned above has prevented psychiatry from being able to study the relationship between patient experience of symptoms and the brain and to augment diagnostic classification systems on this basis. In our view, to the extent that the current DSM avoids the same conceptual problems and necessary anchoring in phenomenology both the clinician and the patients (!), it will continue to lapse into the same unsolvable "metaphysical" problems (mind vs. body, inner vs. outer, self vs. other, history vs. essence, nomothetic vs. idiographic, top-down vs. bottom-up approaches to mental disorder) that previous DSMs have exhibited. To the extent that DSM-III and the following DSMs base their putatively reliable descriptions of mental disorders on everyday language, then folk psychological and other kinds of assumptions, including *metaphysical* assumptions, creep into the classification system [47].

In fact, metaphoric thinking may be an inextricable component in philosophic and scientific thinking in general. Lakoff and Johnson [72] write that we are driven by an "unconscious metaphysics" in our conceptual thinking: "Throughout history, it has been virtually impossible for philosophers to do metaphysics without such metaphors … That is, using unconscious everyday metaphors, philosophers seek to make a noncontradictory choice of conceptual entities defined by these metaphors; then they take these metaphors to be real and then seek out the implications of that choice in an attempt to account for our experience using that metaphysics" (p. 14).

Conclusions

We have not presented empirical evidence to back up our claim of the usefulness of phenomenology in both future diagnostic classification and clinical neuroscience. In several recent studies [73, 74], we have been finding phenomenological and possibly neurobiological similarities between schizophrenia patients' episodic memories of their psychotic experiences and PTSD patients "flashback" memories of their trauma. Both exhibit similar disruption of temporal consciousness and self-experience. Numerous phenomenological authors including Jaspers, Binswanger, Blankenburg, and Conrad have pointed to a loss of context as fundamental to delusion formation both in the original *perceptual* experience and its memory. In both reports of the original experience and its retrieval, there is a temporal shrinking to the present in which the current moment takes precedence over continuity of self-experience. These phenomenological descriptions are in consilience with later aberrant salience models [37].

The phenomenological view conforms with more recent cognitive-neurobiological research that indicates that the "working self," which organizes the psychological present in terms of current goals, event or episodic memory, and autobiographical self-knowledge constrain one another. Coherent self-experience plays a key role in integrating episodic memories into the more enduring self-knowledge: "When the connection between episodic memories and the self becomes disrupted, as occurs following several different types of brain damage... and in certain forms of psychopathological illness, then coherence breaks down and ungrounded delusional versions of the self, divorced from reality, emerge" [75]. Notably, autobiographical memory impairments in established schizophrenia are associated with an altered sense of self [76]. The relationship between phenomenology of delusions, memory and self, and specifically its contribution to more recent clinical neurobiological research is an area which requires further exploration.

The hippocampus and associated structures are involved in the rapid, automatic aspects of context-specific event encoding and retrieval, whereby the creation of lasting event-context memories involves the integration of new information with existing mental frameworks or schemas [77]. Such schemas may be disrupted during acute phases of psychosis in schizophrenia and during those experiences which lead to "flashbacks" in PTSD. Noradrenergic and dopaminergic neuromodulation of systems level consolidation processes may contribute to the selective "salience" of details and thus "patchiness" of those memories related to acute illness in the PTSD and schizophrenia groups and thus the association between disrupted self-experience and episodic memory deficits. The above is admittedly a very provisional and to date sketchy account meant to be more illustrative than definitive. The main point is that it suggestively cuts across the DSM-5 proposed clusters indicating that phenomenology, when practiced rigorously enough and with enough fine-grained detail of patient experience, could lead to different hypotheses and results than current thinking.

Interestingly, the neurologist Josef Parvizi reports that with a certain degree of success, he is able to predict implicated brain areas by the kind of aura or seizure reported by the patient (personal communication to AM, October, 2012). As Akil et al. [78] write: "...starting from a diagnosis and searching broadly for genetic causes that are commonly shared across all affected individuals is not likely to succeed, because a great deal of biological heterogeneity lies at the basis of circuit dysfunction... Given the complexity of neural circuits, there are many possible ways to disrupt them…" Still it has not been investigated how a phenomenology of the patient's subjective experience of symptoms may provide fine-grained analyses that could be linked with very specific neural circuit dysfunction that goes beyond current efforts to separate bottom-up from top-down approaches for DSM-5.

References

1. Hempel CG. Typological methods in the natural and social sciences. In: Aspects of scientific explanation and other essays in the philosophy of science. New York: Free Press; 1965. p. 155–72.
2. Schwartz MA, Wiggins OP. Logical empiricism and psychiatric classification. Compr Psychiatry. 1986;27:101–14.
3. Mayes R, Horwitz A. DSM-III and the revolution in the classification of mental illness. J Hist Behav Sci. 2005;41:249–67.
4. Millon T. Classification in psychopathology: rationale, alternatives, and standards. J Abnorm Psychol. 1991;100:245–61.
5. Williams JBW, Spitzer RL. Research diagnostic criteria and DSM-III. An annotated comparison. Arch Gen Psychiatry. 1982;39:1283–9.
6. Jaspers K. Allgemeine psychopathologie. Berlin: Springer; 1913.
7. Jaspers K. Allgemeine psychopathologie. 4th ed. Berlin: Springer. English edition: General psychopathology [J. Hoenig & M. W. Hamilton, Trans.]. Manchester, UK: Manchester University Press; 1946/1963.
8. Schwartz MA, Wiggins OP. The hegemony of the DSMs. In: Sadler JZ, editor. Descriptions and prescriptions: values, mental disorders, and the DSMs. Baltimore: Johns Hopkins University Press; 2002. p. 199–209.
9. Schwartz MA, Wiggins OP. Typifications. The first step for clinical diagnosis in psychiatry. J Nerv Ment Dis. 1987;175:65–77.
10. Uhlhaas PJ, Mishara AL. Perceptual anomalies in schizophrenia: integrating phenomenology and cognitive neuroscience. Schizophr Bull. 2007;33:142–56.
11. Gadamer, H-G. Truth and method. Second revised edition. [J. Weinsheimer, D. G. Marshall, Trans.]. New York: Continuum; 1993.
12. Damasio AR. The somatic marker hypothesis and the possible functions of the prefrontal cortex. Philos Trans R Soc Lond. 1996;351:1413–20.
13. Mishara AL. Missing links in phenomenological clinical neuroscience? Why we are still not there yet. Curr Opin Psychiatry. 2007;60:559–69.
14. Bransford JD, Brown AL, Cocking RR. How people learn, brain, mind, experience and school. Washington, DC: National Academics Press; 2000.
15. Mishara AL. How can neuroscience inform best teaching practices for training tomorrow's professionals? Seeds for innovation, learning methods for tomorrow. http://www.seedsforinnovation.org/tag/aaron-mishara/.
16. Mezzich J, Snaedal J, Van Weel C, Heath I. Toward person-centered medicine: from disease to patient to person. Mt Sinai J Med. 2010;77:304–6.
17. Schwartz MA, Mishara AL, Wiggins O. The biopsychosocial model is not a straw man: how Jaspers' phenomenology opens the way to a paradigm shift in psychiatry. Existenz. 2011;6(1):17–24. http://www.bu.edu/paideia/existenz/index.html.
18. Mishara AL, Schwartz M. Who's on first? Mental disorders by any other name? Bull Assoc Adv Philos Psychiatry. 2010;17:60–3. http://alien.dowling.edu/~cperring/aapp/bulletin_v_17_2/37.doc.
19. Mishara AL, Schwartz M. Final comment: phenomenology and operationalism: not opposites but mutually in need of one another. Bull Assoc Adv Philos Psychiatry. 2010;17:60–3. http://alien.dowling.edu/~cperring/aapp/bulletin_v_17_2/37.doc.

20. First M. Deconstructing psychosis (February 15–17, 2006) http://www.dsm5.org/research/pages/deconstructingpsychosis(february15-17, 2006).aspx.
21. Conrad K. Die beginnende Schizophrenie. Stuttgart, Germany: Thieme; 1958.
22. Mishara AL. Klaus Conrad (1905–1961): delusional mood, psychosis and beginning schizophrenia. Clinical concept translation-feature. Schizophr Bull. 2010;36:9–13.
23. Ey H. Consciousness: a phenomenological study of being conscious and becoming conscious [J. H. Flodstrom, Trans.]. Bloomington: Indiana University Press; 1978.
24. Hughlings-Jackson J. Lectures on the diagnosis of epilepsy. Br Med J. 1879;1:33–6.
25. Berrios GE, Hauser R. The early development of Kraepelin's ideas on classification: a conceptual history. Psychol Med. 1988;18:813–21.
26. Kraepelin E. Psychiatrie. Ein Lehrbuch fü"r Studirende und Aerzte. Fü"nfte, vollsta"ndig umgearbeitete Auflage. 5. vollsta"ndig umgearbeitete Auflage ed. Leipzig, Germany: Johann Ambrosius Barth; 1896.
27. Heckers S. Bleuler and the neurobiology of schizophrenia. Schizophr Bull. 2011;37:1131–5.
28. Musalek M. [The history of schizophrenias: philosophical roots]. Fortschr Neurol Psychiatr. 2005;73 Suppl 1:S16–24.
29. Shorter E. A historical dictionary of psychiatry. New York, NY: Oxford University Press; 2005.
30. Jablensky A. Diagnosis and revision of the classification systems. In: Gaebel W, editor. Schizophrenia, current science and clinical practice. Hoboken, NJ: Wiley; 2011. p. 10–30.
31. Gaupp R. Über paranoische Veranlagung und abortive Paranoia. Zentralbl Nerven Psychiatr. 1910;33:65–8.
32. Gaupp R. Zur Psychologie des Massenmordes: Hauptlehrer Wagner von Degerloch. Eine kriminalpsyehologisehe und psychiatrische Studie. Berlin: Springer; 1914.
33. Kretchmer E. Der sensitive Beziehungswahn, Ein Beitrag zur Paranoiafrage und zur psychiatrischen Charakterlehre. Berlin: Verlag von Julius Springer; 1918.
34. Freud S. Psychoanalytic notes on an autobiographical account of a case of paranoia (dementia paranoides). In: The standard edition of the complete psychological works of Sigmund Freud. vol. 12. London: Hogarth Press; 1971. p. 3–80.
35. Jaspers K. Eifersuchtswahn, Ein Beitrag zur Frage: "Entwicklung" oder "Prozeß"? Z f ges Neur Psychtr. 1910;11:567–637; Reprinted in Karl Jaspers, Gesammelte Schriften zur Psychopathologie, Berlin: Springer; 1963:85–141.
36. Mishara AL. Kafka, paranoic doubles and the brain: hypnagogic vs. hyper-reflexive models of disruption of self in neuropsychiatric disorders and anomalous conscious states. Philos Ethics Humanit Med. 2010;5:13. http://www.peh-med.com/content/5/1/13.
37. Mishara AL, Fusar-Poli P. The phenomenology and neurobiology of delusions: Jaspers, truman signs, aberrant salience. Schizophr Bull. 2013;39:278–286. doi: 10.1093/schbul/sbs155.
38. Jablensky A. The disease entity in psychiatry: fact or fiction? Epidemiol Psychiatr Sci. 2012;21:255–64. doi:10.1017/S2045796012000339.
39. Andrews G, Goldberg DP, Krueger RF, Carpenter WT, Hyman SE, Sachdev P, et al. Exploring the feasibility of a metastructure for DSMV and ICD11: could it improve utility and validity? Psychol Med. 2009;39:1993–2000. doi:10.1017/S0033291709990250.
40. Hyman SE. Can neuroscience be integrated into the DSM-V? Nat Rev Neurosci. 2007;8: 725–32.
41. Regier DA, Narrow WE, Kuhl EA, Kupfer DJ. The conceptual development of DSM-V. Am J Psychiatry. 2009;166(6):645–50.
42. Kendell RE, Jablensky A. Distinguishing between the validity and utility of psychiatric diagnoses. Am J Psychiatry. 2003;160:4–12.
43. Van Os J. A salience dysregulation syndrome. Br J Psychiatry. 2009;194:101–3.
44. Smith A, Li M, Becker S, Kapur S. Dopamine, prediction error and associative learning: a model-based account. Network. 2006;17:61–84.
45. Mishara AL, Corlett PR. Are delusions biologically adaptive? Salvaging the doxastic shear pin. Behav Brain Sci. 2009;32:530–1.

46. Blankenburg W. Ein Beitrag zum Normproblem. In: Bräutigam W, editor. Medizinisch-psychologische Anthropologie. Darmstadt: Wissenschaftliche Buchgesellschaft; 1980. p. 273–89.
47. Mishara AL. A phenomenological critique of commonsensical assumptions of DSM-III-R: the avoidance of the patient's subjectivity. In: Sadler J, Schwartz MA, Wiggins O, editors. Philosophical perspectives on psychiatric diagnostic classification. Baltimore: Johns Hopkins Series in psychiatry and neuroscience; 1994. p. 129–47.
48. Mishara AL, Schwartz MA. Conceptual analysis of psychiatric approaches: phenomenology, psychopathology and classification. Curr Opin Psychiatry. 1995;6:312–7.
49. Mishara A, Schwartz M. Psychopathology in the light of emergent trends in the philosophy of consciousness, neuropsychiatry and phenomenology. Curr Opin Psychiatry. 1997;10:383–9.
50. Mishara AL, Schwartz M. Altered states of consciousness as paradoxically healing: an embodied social neuroscience perspective. In: Cardeña E, Winkelman M, editors. Altering consciousness: a multidisciplinary perspective, vol. II. New York: Plenum Press; 2011. p. 327–53.
51. Viktor von Weizsäcker: Der Gestaltkreis. Theorie der Einheit von Wahrnnehmen und Bewegen 4. Aufl. Stuttgart, Georg Thieme Verlag; 1950.
52. Bridgeman B, Hoover M. Processing spatial layout by perception and sensorimotor interaction. Q J Exp Psychol. 2008;61:851–9. doi:10.1080/17470210701623712.
53. Ramsperger AG. Objects perceived and objects known. J Philos. 1940;37:291–7.
54. Mishara AL, Fusar-Poli P. The phenomenology and neurobiology of delusions: Jaspers, tru- man signs, aberrant salience. Schizophr Bull. 2013;39:278–286. doi: 10.1093/schbul/sbs155.
55. Blankenburg W. First steps toward a 'psychopathology of common sense' [Aaron L. Mishara, trans.]. Philos Psychiatr Psychol. 2001;8:303–15. Originally published in 1969.
56. Fiske ST. Social beings, core motives in social psychology. 2nd ed. Hoboken, NJ: Wiley; 2010.
57. De Dreu CKW, Greer LL, Van Kleef GA, Shalvi S, Handgraaf MJJ. Oxytocin promotes ethnocentrism. Proc Natl Acad Sci USA. 2011;108:1262–6.
58. Jaspers K. Psychologie der Weltanschauungen. 6th unchanged edition. Berlin: Springer; 1920/1990.
59. Heider F. The psychology of interpersonal relations. New Jersey: Hillsdale; 1958.
60. Pronin E. Perception and misperception of bias in human judgment. Trends Cogn Sci. 2007;11:37–43.
61. Jones EE, Nisbett RE. The actor and the observer: divergent perceptions of the causes of behavior. Morristown, NJ: General Learning Press; 1971.
62. Decety J. A social cognitive neuroscience model of empathy. In: Harmon Jones E, Winkelman P, editors. Social neuroscience, integrating biological and psychological explanations of behavior. New York: The Guilford Press; 2007. p. 246–70.
63. Wiggins O, Schwartz MA. Karl Jaspers. In: Embree L., et al., editors. Encyclopedia of phenomenology. Dordrecht, Netherlands: Kluwer Academic; 1997. p. 371–6.
64. Jablensky A. Categories, dimensions and prototypes: critical issues for psychiatric classification. Psychopathology. 2005;38:201–5.
65. Schwartz MA, Wiggins OP, Norko MA. Prototypes, ideal types and personality disorders: the return to classical phenomenology. In: Livesley, editor. The DSM-IV personality disorders. New York: The Guilford Press; 1995. p. 420–32.
66. Kendler KS. An historical framework for psychiatric nosology. Psychol Med. 2009;39: 1935–41. doi:10.1017/S0033291709005753.
67. Kendler KS, First MB. Alternative futures for the DSM revision process: iteration v. paradigm shift. Br J Psychiatry. 2010;197:263–5.
68. Kupfer DJ, Regier DA. Neuroscience, clinical evidence, and the future of psychiatric classification in DSM-5. Am J Psychiatry. 2011;168(7):672–4.
69. Regier DA, Kuhl EA, Kupfer DJ, McNulty JP. Patient involvement in the development of DSM-V. Psychiatry. 2010;73(4):308–10.
70. Miller R, Frese FJ, Chadwick PK. Reflections from within. Three stories from inside psychosis. In: Mishara AL, Corlett P, Fletcher P, Kranjec A, Schwartz MA, editors. Phenomenological

neuropsychiatry, how patient experience bridges clinic with clinical neuroscience. New York: Springer; 2013.

71. Mishara AL, Schwartz MA. The DSMs: wedge between clinician and clinical researcher? In: Phillips J, Frances A, editors. The six most essential questions in psychiatric diagnosis: a pluralogue. With commentaries by Michael Cerullo, John Chardavoyne, Michael First, Nassir Ghaemi, Gary Greenberg, Andrew Hinderleiter, Warren Kinghorn, Steven Labello, Elliott Martin, Aaron Mishara, Joel Paris, Joseph Pierre, Ronald Pies, Harold Pincus, Douglas Porter, Claire Pouncey, Michael Schwartz, Thomas Szasz, Jerome Wakefield, Scott Waterman, Owen Whooley, Peter Zachar. Philos Ethics Humanit Med (PEHM). PubMed Central Open Access Journal; 2012. www.peh-med.com/content/7/1/9.

72. Lakoff G, Johnson M. Philosophy in the flesh. The embodied mind and its challenge to western thought. New York: Basic Books; 1999.

73. Mishara AL, Clews K, Bonnemann C. Episodic memory and experience of self in PTSD and schizophrenia: common neurobiological mechanisms? In: Slide presentation in the nano symposium: human long-term memory, medial temporal lobe. New Orleans: Society for Neuroscience Conference, Oct 2012.

74. Mishara AL, Thorrud K, Bonnemann C. Phenomenology of self in delusions of reference in beginning schizophrenia. Schizophr Bull. 2011;37 Suppl 1:9 (abstract)

75. Conway MA, Singer JA, Taginia A. The self and autobiographical memory: correspondence and coherence. Soc Cogn. 2004;22(5):491–529.

76. Bennouna-Greene M, Berna F, Conway MA, Rathbone CJ, Vidailhet P, Danion J-M. Self-images and related autobiographical memories in schizophrenia. Conscious Cogn. 2012; 21: 247–57.

77. Tse D, Langston RF, Kakeyama M, Bethus I, Spooner PA, Wood ER, et al. Schemas and memory consolidation. Science. 2007;316:76–82.

78. Akil H, Brenner S, Kandel E, et al. The future of psychiatric research: genomes and neural circuits. Science. 2010;327:1580–1.

Chapter 10
The Conceptual Status of DSM-5 Diagnoses

James Phillips

Introduction: Why Question the Conceptual Status of DSM-5 Diagnoses?

This chapter begins by asking: why question the conceptual status of DSM diagnoses? Or still, why now? The answer is clear. The question arises at this point because, in the aftermath of DSM-III and DSM-IV, and in context of the development of DSM-5, we have experienced a crisis of confidence in the validity of our psychiatric diagnoses. Do the diagnoses accurately reflect real psychiatric illnesses from which real people suffer? Or to be more specific, do using the appropriate diagnostic criteria and giving someone a diagnosis of, say, schizophrenia guarantee us that there is a real condition, schizophrenia, and that this person suffers from it?

I will move to the reasons for the crisis of confidence in a moment, but first we need a preliminary clarification. The question as to the conceptual status of DSM diagnoses in fact involves two questions: what Claire Pouncey has distinguished as questions of epistemological and ontological realism [1]. The title of this chapter raises the first, epistemological, question: do our diagnoses give us an accurate window into psychiatric disorders? But this question hides a second, that of ontological realism: what are psychiatric disorders? We can see this double question in the title of Robins and Guze's seminal 1970 article, "Establishment of diagnostic validity in psychiatric illness: Its application to schizophrenia" [2]. Robins and Guze didn't ask the second question. They assumed the reality of schizophrenia. Their concern was to diagnosis it correctly. (And of course they were writing during an era of overdiagnosis of schizophrenia in the United States) But we no longer share their confidence in the reality of the conditions we name with our diagnostic categories. For that reason this chapter includes the question named in the chapter title,

J. Phillips, MD (✉)
Department of Psychiatry, Yale School of Medicine, 88 Noble Avenue,
New Haven, CT 06460, USA
e-mail: james.phillips@yale.edu

J. Paris and J. Phillips (eds.), *Making the DSM-5: Concepts and Controversies*,
DOI 10.1007/978-1-4614-6504-1_10, © Springer Science+Business Media New York 2013

the conceptual status of diagnostic categories, and in addition the question hidden under the first, the conceptual status of psychiatric disorders themselves.

So let us now turn to the reasons for the breakdown of confidence. For this we begin with Robins and Guze, who, along with colleagues developing their approach [3, 4], set the stage for the predicament in which we find ourselves 42 years later. In their 1970 article Robins and Guze set five criteria or standards of validity (called "phases of validity" in the article), in psychiatric diagnosis. Ten years later, with the publication of DSM-III, diagnostic categories were defined operationally with diagnostic criteria. The primary concern of Robert Spitzer and the other authors of DSM-III was to establish reliability in psychiatric diagnosis—the assurance that clinicians and researchers in different settings would be talking about the same condition when they used a particular diagnostic label. The assumption of everyone involved in the construction of DSM-III was that in the research that would follow, and be aided by, DSM-III, the diagnostic categories would gradually meet the validity standards set by Robins and Guze. A well-defined DSM-III diagnosis would be proven to represent a real psychiatric disorder. The goals of epistemological and ontological realism would be achieved. Regier and colleagues summarized this expectation.

> The expectation of Robins and Guze was that each clinical syndrome described in the Feighner criteria, RDC, and DSM-III would ultimately be validated by its separation from other disorders, common clinical course, genetic aggregation in families, and further differentiation by future laboratory tests—which would now include anatomical and functional imaging, molecular genetics, pathophysiological variations, and neuropsychological testing. To the original validators Kendler added differential response to treatment, which could include both pharmacological and psychotherapeutic interventions [5].

The great shock of the past 40 years has been that these goals have not been achieved. And of course, if there is no validity, what good is reliability? If we can reliably define a particular disease, but there is no evidence that the disease actually exists, what good is our reliable diagnosis?

Status of Robins/Guze Validity Criteria

It is worthwhile reviewing briefly the Robins/Guze criteria, along with the current status of clinical experience and psychiatric research. The five standards (or "phases" in their language) were clinical description, laboratory studies, delimitation from other disorders, follow-up studies, and family studies. The sixth standard proposed by Kendler in 1990 was differential response to treatment [6].

1. Clinical description. This includes symptoms aggregating into syndromes, along with other information involved in the common description. Clinical work with the DSM categories has shown a great heterogeneity of presentation, thus defeating the criterion that a valid category should present a uniformly described syndrome. Hyman notes how this has led to a plethora of NOS diagnoses: "…a significant fraction of patients do not fit the highly specified criteria of named disorders.

In this case, the rigidity of operationalized diagnostic criteria, based on phenomenology, trades interrater reliability for ability to capture the true heterogeneity of clinical populations" [7].

This phenomenon of heterogeneous presentation should not be a surprise, as it is common in the rest of medicine, where the same disease may present in different ways, and a similar presentation may represent different diseases. For instance, syphilis and streptococcus may each present in a variety of ways (same disease, different presentations), and shortness of breath may represent CHF, pneumonia, or COPD (same presentation, different diseases). The reason this is not a problem for general medicine is that the labeling of something as a disease is not dependent on the clinical presentation, as in psychiatry. For the rest of medicine there are biological markers, as well as physiological and anatomical abnormalities, to confirm the validity of the diagnosis. In this regard psychiatry is in the place of the rest of medicine of 100 years ago. Further, we can note in retrospect that "clinical description" was a poor choice of validator by Robins and Guze and that, based on the rest of medicine, it was bound to fail.

2. Laboratory studies. The most striking example of the failure of laboratory studies is that we still do not have a clear biological marker for any of our DSM categories. In the words of Kupfer and colleagues, "Despite many proposed candidates, not one laboratory marker has been found to be specific in identifying any of the DSM-defined syndromes" [8]. And we have to add that current work in neuroscience, neuroimaging, and genetics has not led to clear patterns that match up with the DSM categories [9–11]. Probably the most alarming findings are in genetic studies, where the mismatch between genetic patterns and DSM categories has become quite clear [9, 10]. What now seems obvious is that the science is not falling into place because the DSM categories do not represent distinct diseases— or, in the language of genetics, do not represent real phenotypes.

3. Delimitation from other disorders. With this criterion Robins and Guze recognized that the first two criteria might allow for two disorders to overlap with similar description and laboratory findings, and that we would need a way to distinguish them. In strong contrast to meeting this standard, DSM-IV has been plagued with high comorbidity, along with fuzzy boundaries between categories and the use of NOS diagnoses [12–14]. To quote Hyman once again: "Finally, the frequency of comorbidity among DSM-IV diagnoses is so great as to suggest underlying problems with the current classification. Certainly, an individual may have more than one illness; for instance, the presence of mania may elevate the risk of substance use disorders. However, the high rates of comorbidity…raise the question of whether too many disorders have been stipulated and whether the categorical approach is always the right one" [7].

4. Follow-up study. The authors acknowledge that this is not a strong criterion, inasmuch as the same condition could have variable outcomes. That has of course been found to be the case with major disorders such as schizophrenia and bipolar disorder.

5. Family study. The authors argued for this as a strong criterion, and indeed, identical twin studies have shown family aggregation for many conditions.

The problem is that family studies have shown both a higher familial incidence of the condition of the target patient, but also a high incidence of other psychiatric disorders [15, 16]. And genetic studies have shown similar genetic patterns in a variety of conditions [7, 8, 17]. Thus, although family and genetic research have demonstrated strong evidence of family clustering and genetic heritability, they have not supported the notion of the DSM-IV categories as clear phenotypes.

6. Differential response to treatment. In 1990 Kenneth Kendler proposed a sixth criterion for validity [6]. Unfortunately, clinical experience over the past 20 years has moved rather dramatically against this criterion. Rather than classes of psychopharmacologic agents matching up with particular diagnoses, we have moved into an era of pharmacologic promiscuity in which many agents are being found to be effective for a variety of disorders (e.g., neuroleptics effective as mood stabilizers, SSRIs effective for a great variety of conditions).

If the DSM diagnostic categories have failed to meet the Robins/Guze standards of validity, we are forced to ask, what are these diagnostic categories? Are they anything real? This question was the subject of extended by discussion by Allen Frances and others in a series of articles [18–20]. Frances' position has been that the categories are constructs that aim to describe real psychiatric disorders in the real world, but that as constructs they are vulnerable to failure on the dual fronts of epistemological and ontological realism. That is: (1) the construct may do a poor job of describing the disorder it intends to describe; and (2) the particular disorder may not really exist in the manner suggested by the diagnostic category. If, for instance, it emerges that what we label as schizophrenia and bipolar disorder turn out to be different presentations of a single disorder, our categories will have done a poor job at describing psychiatric reality, and psychiatric reality will prove to be different from that suggested in the diagnostic categories. The epistemology and the ontology will have proved to be wrong. Whatever the value of this particular example, it is the case that our diagnostic constructs have not held up under scientific scrutiny. They do not appear to describe the reality of psychiatric illness. None of this should be taken to suggest that psychiatric illness does not exist. The point is rather that our diagnostic constructs have not done a very good job of reflecting than that illness.

The DSM-5 Response

What has been the DSM-5 response to the crisis of validity in the DSM categories? In an early statement in the 2002 white papers published as *A Research Agenda for DSM-V*, DSM-5 leaders clearly recognized the problem.

> In the more than 30 years since the introduction of the Feighner criteria by Robins and Guze, which eventually led to DSM-III, the goal of validating these syndromes and discovering common etiologies has remained elusive. Despite many proposed candidates, not one laboratory marker has been found to be specific in identifying any of the DSM-defined

syndromes. Epidemiologic and clinical studies have shown extremely high rates of comorbidities among the disorders, undermining the hypothesis that the syndromes represent distinct etiologies. Furthermore, epidemiologic studies have shown a high degree of short-term diagnostic instability for many disorders. With regard to treatment, lack of treatment specificity is the rule rather than the exception [8].

The authors' response to this crisis was a vague appeal for a "paradigm shift."

All these limitations in the current diagnostic paradigm suggest that research exclusively focused on refining the DSM-defined syndromes may never be successful in uncovering their underlying etiologies. For that to happen, an as yet unknown paradigm shift may need to occur. Therefore, another important goal of this volume is to transcend the limitations of the current DSM paradigm and to encourage a research agenda that goes beyond our current ways of thinking to attempt to integrate information from a wide variety of sources and technologies (p. 19).

In the 2002 *A Research Agenda*, the publication of DSM-5 was announced for 2010. It is now scheduled for May, 2013. In the past 10 years we have not seen the much-heralded paradigm shift—for the obvious reason that the science is not in place to effect such a major change. In the face of the failure to achieve that goal, we have seen a number of other maneuvers on the part of the DSM-5 leadership. One has been endless refining of the DSM categories, a strategy that the above quote declared a nonstarter for making serious progress in uncovering underlying etiologies.

Another effort to accomplish change in DSM-5 is a general restructuring of the manual. One proposal has been to collapse the first three axes into one axis, bringing DSM-5 more into conformity with ICD-10. A second proposal has been to reorganize the diagnostic categories into a more logical scientific hierarchy. Both of these proposals will presumably be implemented in DSM-5.

Still another effort to accomplish change with DSM-5 involves the introduction of new DSM categories. One was the Pre-psychosis Risk Syndrome, later renamed Attenuated Psychosis Syndrome. This new category generated significant controversy because of its faulty scientific status and has recently been relegated to Section III appendix at the back of the manual, a section designated for proposed disorders needing "further study." Other innovations moved to Section III are Mixed Anxiety Depressive Disorder, Hypersexual Disorder, and Paraphilic Coercive Disorder, the latter because of its obvious potential use as a psychiatric diagnosis for the garden-variety rapist. These decisions have presumably been determined or influenced by the Scientific Review Committee, appointed by the APA Board of Trustees to oversee changes proposed by the DSM-5 Work Groups. The work of the SRC is not made available for outside scrutiny. One controversial innovation that has thus far survived SRC inspection is Disruptive Mood Dysregulation Disorder, a disorder that is diagnosed between the ages of 6 and 18, is characterized by temper outbursts, and is presumably DSM-5's response to what has been perceived as an overdiagnosis of bipolar disorder in children.

In view of the failure to achieve the desired paradigm shift with DSM-5, the change proposal considered most important by the DSM-5 community has been the introduction of dimensional measures. In 2009 Regier and colleagues emphasized the importance of dimensional measures for DSM-5:

> The single most important precondition for moving forward to improve the clinical and scientific utility of DSM-V will be the incorporation of simple dimensional measures for assessing syndromes within broad diagnostic categories and supraordinate dimensions that cross current diagnostic boundaries. Thus, we have decided that one, if not the major, difference between DSM-IV and DSM-V will be the more prominent use of dimensional measures in DSM-V [5].

The underlying principal is clear: if the diagnostic categories do hold up as valid phenotypes, with the consequences of fuzzy boundaries and large-scale comorbidity, this problem can be somewhat rectified by viewing the categories as spectrum disorders in which poor boundaries and comorbidities are expected rather than disturbing. The original proposal was for "cross-cutting" measures for every patient assessment, along with individual severity measures for every disorder. The cross-cutting measures would assess anxiety, depression, and other candidate symptoms for every patient. These measures have disappeared from the DSM-5 web site without explanation, presumably because they impose an intolerable burden on the examiner and for that reason would almost certainly not be used. Many of the severity measures have also disappeared from the DSM-5 web site. A final blow to the extensive use of dimensional measures in DSM-5 was a vote by the APA General Assembly in May, 2012, to remove them from the front of the manual. The dimensional measures associated with the personality disorders were also voted out. One look at them would make it clear to the reader that they also are so burdensome and time-consuming for the evaluator that they would almost certainly be ignored.

What is striking in this review of DSM-5 innovations is not just that the proposed paradigm shift is missing but that the new diagnostic manual will have so little of substance to replace it. To complete the review, we look at the recent statement by Kupfer and Regier.

> A logical extension of those discussions, as detailed in our *Research Agenda* [1] articles, is the Research Domain Criteria (RDoC) initiative recently launched by the National Institute of Mental Health (NIMH)...This NIMH objective is consistent with our research planning conferences and conclusions, which underscored our commitment to examining evidence from neurobiology and assessing the readiness of proposed revisions for DSM-5. We are pleased with the work on RDoC that is being undertaken, and we believe this initiative will be very informative for subsequent versions: DSM-5.1, DSM-5.2, and beyond...It is important to emphasize that DSM-5 does not represent a radical departure from the past, nor does it represent a radical separation from the goals of the RDoC [21].

The DSM-5 embrace of the Research Domain Criteria (RDoC) project is striking in that the project was developed specifically outside the boundaries of the DSM categories, and indeed in recognition of the fact that the DSM categories and diagnostic criteria represent a blind alley in research into the etiology of psychiatric disorders. The irony in this linkage of DSM-5 to the RDoC research findings is that the DSM-5 architects are now presenting the RDoC effectively as the accomplishment and salvation of DSM-5.

The Way Forward in Analyzing DSM-5 Categories

It should be clear from the above that the DSM categories are in a state of conceptual bankruptcy, and further, that the DSM-5 salvage job will accomplish little beyond requiring us to purchase and learn to use a new manual. It has always been an axiom of the DSMs that revisions and new additions primarily serve the interests of the clinicians. In the above cited article Kupfer and Regier continue this fantasy invoking their "philosophy that DSM-5 remains first and foremost a tool for clinicians" [21].

In what follows I propose to get a further grasp on the conceptual status of DSM categories (and psychiatric disorders) by analyzing them with two tools from the philosophy of science: natural-kind analysis and complexity theory.

Natural-Kind Analysis

One way to get a further perspective on this question of the DSM categories and the nature of psychiatric illness is through what is called natural-kind analysis. The latter refers to the effort to classify the things of the world in a realistic manner that does not depend on human judgment. A cow is a natural kind, a unicorn is not. You may come across a specimen in the real world and declare it to belong to the natural kind, cow. You won't find anything fitting the natural kind, unicorn. Writing about natural kinds, Ian Hacking remarks: "The canonical examples have been: water, sulphur, horse, tiger, lemon, multiple sclerosis, heat and the color yellow. What an indifferent bunch!" [22]. Hacking includes everything that can be classified, but in a more strict sense a natural kind is considered to have an essential structure that can be described by necessary and sufficient conditions. For instance, if something has an atomic weight of 79, that something is gold; if another thing has a molecular structure of H_2O, that thing is water. In both cases the thing in the world meets necessary and sufficient conditions for being gold or water. John Locke provided an early description of the strict sense of natural kinds with his distinction between real and nominal essences. The latter category represents our casual manner of classifying things, as in the Hacking quote above. A real essence would be defined in terms of its microstructure. In making this distinction Locke anticipated our modern tendency to define strict natural-kind status in terms of the reductionist language of physics. The examples of gold and water are characteristic of this tendency.

Among philosophers of science there is a fundamental divide between strict natural-kind theorists as just described who assign natural-kind status only to entities that can be defined by essential properties and necessary and sufficient conditions, and other theorists who take a more inclusivist view of natural kinds, incorporating our great variety of ways to classify the world. John Dupré argues in

The Disorder of Things for the latter approach: "This thesis is an assertion of the extreme diversity of the contents of the world. There are countless kinds of things, I maintain, subject each to its own characteristic behavior and interactions" [23]. From this perspective there is a scale of natural kindness: something may be a natural kind in a strong or weak sense.

In a strict sense all medical and psychiatric conditions would be judged as not natural kinds because in every case designating something as a disease involves a human value judgment. A broken bone may be an objective, strong natural kind, but declaring the broken bone an ailment involves a value judgment that does not inhere in the bone.

In thinking about medical and psychiatric conditions, however, it is more useful to sort out the world of illness with degrees of natural kindness. For instance, HIV infection can be defined with the necessary and sufficient condition of a positive test; Huntington's disease can be defined with the necessary and sufficient condition of the Huntington gene HTT. These are relatively strong natural kinds. On the other hand, migraine is defined by clinical evaluation; schizophrenia and major depression are defined by symptoms and diagnostic criteria. These latter three are all quite weak natural kinds compared to HIV or Huntington's disease, and even more so compared to gold or water. There are no necessary and sufficient conditions for calling something migraine, schizophrenia, or major depression. Indeed, if schizophrenia, for instance, turns out be not one disease but rather a cluster of diseases, it may be a natural kind only in a very weak sense.[1]

In the discussions referred to above Allen Frances and others have argued that DSM diagnostic categories are constructs that point to real psychiatric illness but may not represent it accurately. This is another way of arguing that the categories are weak natural kinds. They are a way of dividing and classifying the world of mental illness, but not a way in which diagnoses will describe necessary and sufficient conditions of entities that exist in the real world. The fact, for instance, that we don't have any biological markers to confirm our diagnoses points to the weak natural-kind status of these diagnoses. In general medicine, in contrast, a condition like diabetes may not meet natural-kind necessary and sufficient conditions in the manner of the element, gold, but the multiple physiological and anatomical markers of the disease certainly place it higher on the natural-kind scale than, say, schizophrenia.

If we accept this view that psychiatric disorders are weak natural kinds that do not meet any standard of necessary and sufficient conditions, it will follow that they may be grouped in different ways to satisfy different strategies. Often the strategy is an effort to achieve a more scientific, natural-kind status. The authors of DSM-5, for instance, argue that there is evidence of a fear/avoidance neural circuitry

---

[1] Peter Zachar has covered much of this ground in his The Practical Kinds Model as a Pragmatist Theory of Classification [32]. He limits the term natural kind for those entities I am calling strong natural kinds.

dysfunction that warrants grouping PTSD, panic/agoraphobia, social anxiety, and specific phobias together, and distinguishing them from other anxiety disorders such as generalized anxiety disorder, obsessive-compulsive disorder, and impulse control disorders [21].

Such grouping and regrouping of psychiatric disorders may seem arbitrary, and of course it is. At this point in time all psychiatric disorders are weak natural kinds, albeit some weaker than others. As weak natural kinds, we will group them as it seems useful for whatever purpose we have in mind. Our groupings will start with the commonalities—the natural-kind status—that we do find, and our decisions as to how to proceed from there will depend on what we find most useful for what we are trying to accomplish. While it is obvious that some groupings will be useful than others, we need to bear in mind that all groupings are provisional [24], and many display traces of their historical contingency [25].

For an example of psychiatric disorders as weak natural kinds, let's imagine that the current category of schizophrenia, proves, as seems likely, to include a variety of conditions with different genetic patterns, different endophenotypes, different outcomes, and so forth. For a variety of reasons we may decide to retain the super-category, schizophrenia, or to break it up into five, ten, or fifty separate conditions. There will be no one, right answer to the question, how to group or regroup all the individuals that now fall under that category. Which of course is to say that we don't expect any of the possible outcomes to enjoy the status of strong natural kind with necessary and sufficient conditions like those of Huntington's disease. A classification based on endophenotypes, such as the RDoC enterprise (to be discussed below), might claim stronger scientific, natural-kind status, and for that reason might make a claim for priority in the reclassification of schizophrenia. But that classification might be very unwieldy as well as less desirable for other reasons. At this point we have no idea how we will want to classify today's schizophrenics in 10 years.

Or imagine that we decide to remove the paraphilias from the diagnostic manual for a variety of pragmatic and political/societal reasons. They will still maintain a weak natural-kind status as a way to classify these personality types, but for reasons other than scientific ones will no longer be members of the diagnostic manual. And it's hard to imagine any scientific finding that will move the paraphilias into a stronger natural-kind status requiring us to declare them psychiatric diseases that *must* remain in the manual.

I referred above to the NIMH RDoC project, and I conclude this discussion of natural kinds with that project. As mentioned above, the developers of the project recognize that the effort to validate the DSM categories as real phenotypes has failed. The RDoC work is premised on the assumptions that (1) psychiatric disorders originate in disruptions or malfunctions of neural circuitry, and (2) that specific circuitry malfunctions can be linked to specific cognitive and behavioral abnormalities. Their presumption is further that the genetic basis of these malfunctions may be more clearly defined than the complex patterns associated with DSM categories. The target dysfunctions of the RDoC research would then represent genuine endophenotypes. Of course it remains to be seen how successful the RDoC project will be, and whether it will translate into a more scientific nosology than the current DSM. Again, as mentioned above, the authors of DSM-5 hold out the promise that the RDoC research will be integrated into DSM-5 and will effectively save it [21]. In the context of natural-kind analysis, it seems at least possible that the RDoC dysfunctions will enjoy stronger natural-kind status than the DSM categories. What remains completely unclear is in what manner they will be used and how they will fold into a usable nosology. Since the target dysfunctions will be narrow, delimited, endophenotypic dysfunctions that might be one aspect of one or more diagnostic categories, they are a perfect example of the phenomenon of multiple ways of dividing and classifying psychopathology.

Complexity Theory

In the above analysis I examined psychiatric diagnoses and disorders from the perspective of natural-kind analysis. The conclusion of that examination was that psychiatric disorders are weak natural kinds. We now approach psychiatric conditions from a different perspective, complexity theory. Complexity theory and the related chaos theory have been described in a variety of way. For this discussion I will follow the relatively simple and straightforward approach to complexity developed by Bechtel and Richardson [26].

Bechtel and Richardson analyze complex behavior through a process of decomposition and localization. In this process a system is decomposed into its parts and then understood in terms of how the parts work in producing the whole system or mechanism. They describe three levels of such mechanistic explanation. The first, termed aggregative, describes a system in which each part has its task, and the functioning of the whole can be understood in terms of the components working together, each contributing its specific function. The working of ordinary machines like clocks and automobiles can be understood in this bottom-up, aggregative analysis. Each component part can be examined as a separate entity that, together with the other parts, produces the functioning mechanism. This process is highly reductive. Take the machine apart and you have the assembly of parts. Reassemble them correctly and you have the working clock or automobile.

Biological systems virtually never permit of such reductive analysis. They involve further levels of complexity than the clock or automobile, and Bechtel and Richardson describe two further levels of complexity to accommodate biologic systems. With each of the two further levels, a particular part cannot be analyzed in isolation from other parts. What a part is and how it works is determined by its relation to the other parts and to the whole mechanism. "Some machines, however, are much more complex: one component may affect and be affected by several others, with a cascading effect; or there may be significant feedback from 'later' to 'earlier' stages. In the latter case, what is functionally dependent becomes unclear. *Interaction* among components becomes critical. Mechanisms of this latter kind are *complex systems*...In such cases, attempting to understand the operation of the entire machine by following the activities in each component in a brute force manner is liable to be futile" (p. 18).

Analysis of complex systems proceeds through an interplay of analysis and synthesis, bottom-up and top-down approaches. The whole is understood in terms of the parts, but the parts are also understood in terms of each other and of the whole. In the simpler form of complex system termed *component system*, the component parts can still be studied independently, despite the fact that their actual functioning will depend on the total organization of the system. In the more complex *integrated system* the component parts lose their independence and can only be studied as components of the integrated system. What they are and how they work will change with the changing organization of the whole system.

Virtually all biologic systems are complex, as are virtually all diseases. Although a disease like Huntington's disease might be described as a *component* system of limited complexity, with straightforward Mendelian causality, many medical diseases and all psychiatric disorders may be better described as *integrated* systems. They follow Bechtel and Richardson's principle that "In *integrated systems*, systemic organization is significantly involved in determining constituent functions" (p. 20).

The problem we face in recognizing psychiatric disorders as complex, integrated systems is that it is extremely difficult to study them in this manner. Any particular factor playing a role in the production of the disorder is affected by all the other factors at play. Imagine a putative condition with a background of multiple genetic loci and multiple epigenetic factors, as well as personality, psychological, and environmental factors playing etiological roles in the end-result disorder—and any one of these various etiological factors possibly affecting the functioning of any of the others, and you have a picture of almost unimaginable complexity.

One example of such complexity is the RDoC project just discussed. The research design of RDoC is represented by a matrix with rows and columns. The rows contain five major domains of functioning, each domain containing more specific constructs. These are the units that are expected to be related to dysfunctions of neurocircuitry and that may represent genuine endophenotypes. The domains and the specific constructs are also expected to match up with symptoms found in the usual diagnostic categories. The five domains are the Negative Valence Systems, with constructs for fear, distress, and aggression; the Positive Valence Systems, with constructs for reward seeking and learning and habit formation; the Cognitive Systems domain, with constructs for attention, perception, working memory/executive function, long-term memory, and cognitive control; the Systems for Social Process domain, with constructs for separation fear, facial expression regulation, behavioral inhibition, and emotional regulation; and the Arousal/Regulatory Systems domain, with constructs for phenomena involved in sleep and wakefulness.

The columns in the matrix represent the ways in which the domain constructs can be studied. The list of columns includes genes, molecules, cells, circuits, physiology, behavior, and self-report. Of course in this list priority is given to circuits, as the central goal of the project is to relate the domain constructs to dysfunctions in neurocircuitry.

It is not difficult to imagine the difficulties in working with the RDoC as an integrated, complex system. Imagine a discrete attentional problem falling under the Cognitive Systems domain. The RDoC goal would be to associate this behavioral abnormality with a specific circuitry dysfunction and a discrete, endophenogenetic pattern. But the reality might turn out to be several genetic loci converging on this deficit, all affected by epigenetic factors, as well as several neurocircuitry dysfunctions converging on the deficit. Further, the factors represented by columns other than the circuitry column may in various ways affect the emergence of the deficit, all of course also affecting one another. Finally, the target deficit may play a role in several of the current diagnostic categories. In face of this complexity, it's difficult to imagine how such a deficit would be incorporated into a nosological system.

For another example of psychiatric diagnoses and disorders as complex systems, I invoke the work of Kenneth Kendler, psychiatry's premier researcher on the causation of psychiatric illnesses. Kendler has presented a mixed picture in the matter of complexity, arguing strongly for a complexity, decomposition-reassembly, approach to psychiatric etiology [27], and conducting his research in a manner that combines aggregative and integrated styles of analysis. In two articles on developmental models for major depression in women and men, Kendler and colleagues developed the models through the analysis of multiple risk factors, seen both as direct causal agents and as interacting, mutually influencing causal factors [28, 29]. In these studies the authors demonstrate interacting risk factors, one predicting and correlating with another. At the same time they recognize the limitations of these studies in dealing with the full complexity of the multiple factors: "… the models we employed assumed that multiple independent variables act additively and linearly in their impact on a dependent variable. This is unlikely to be true for the etiology of major depression. Although we could have included interactions in our model, the analysis and subsequent interpretation of the very large number of such possible interactions among these variables is daunting" [28].

In his recent "The Dappled Nature of Causes of Psychiatric Illness: Replacing the Organic-functional/hardware-software Dichotomy with Empirically Based Pluralism" [30], Kendler acknowledges his aggregative approach ("Furthermore, for pragmatic reasons, I initially assume an independence of difference-makers that does not exist in nature") (p. 379) and then analyzes the respective variance of multiple causal factors for schizophrenia, major depression, and alcohol dependence in an additive manner. For each of the three conditions he divides the total variance in causal liability into 11 factors (molecular genetic, molecular neuroscience, systems neuroscience, aggregate genetic effects, miscellaneous biological influences, neuropsychology, personality/cognitive, trauma exposure, social, political, and cultural). For each condition he presents a graph showing the percent of variance attributable to each of the 11 factors, totaling 100 %. The study is an elegant example of the empirical pluralism he espouses, as well as of the possibility of still doing valuable research within the confines of the DSM categories. On the other hand, as acknowledged by Kendler himself, it is research in the aggregative mode, with no effort to deal with the complexity of the causal variables—of the multiple ways in which each factor may influence the role of the others. He ends the article with a further statement of this limitation.

> The results of the empirically based pluralistic analysis of the causes of SZ, MD and AD reinforce the conclusions from a prior essay that the commonly expressed wish to develop an etiologically based nosology for psychiatric disorders is deeply problematic. Psychiatric disorders are a result of multiple etiological processes impacting on many different levels and often further intertwined by mediational and moderational interactions between levels. It is not possible a priori to identify one privileged level that can unambiguously be used as the basis for developing a nosologic system. My call for an empirically based pluralism does not reflect pessimism about the future of research in the etiology of psychiatric disorders. Surely, they are stunningly complex. But having overly simplified views of them, often ideologically driven, has only hampered our field. Following methods of decomposition and reassembly, progress has been made in the scientific understanding of very complex systems. Having a realistic view of the causal landscapes of psychiatric disorders can only help (p. 385).

We can take two lessons from Kendler's experience. The first is that research into psychiatric disorders as complex systems will be very difficult. The second is that the research will involve decisions as to which factors, levels of analysis, etc., to prioritize. The prioritizing of one over the other will result in a different picture of the respective disorder. And of course now we are back with the issues of natural-kind analysis—different manners of sorting the field of psychopathology, each potentially equally legitimate, and choices made to serve particular ends.

Conclusion

We can draw three conclusions from this combination of natural-kind and complexity analysis. The first is that complexity analysis leads us to a curious realization. If we imagine a future in which we will have a comprehensive grasp of the factors contributing to psychiatric disorder in all their complexity, we have to assume that no two individuals will have exactly the same causal picture. The Robins/Guze notion of two individuals having the same disorder because they share the same disorder phenotype will, technically, not be realized. Oddly, in a very strict sense every individual with psychiatric illness will have his or her own unique causal picture and his own disorder.

The second conclusion follows from natural-kind analysis and is the corrective of the dilemma created by the first conclusion. In the manner described by natural-kind analysis, it will be our decision where and how to set the dividing lines in our effort to develop a useful nosology. In the vast, complex world of psychopathology, we will decide what are the useful groupings for the purpose at hand. To take examples with which we are already familiar, we might decide that, *for research purposes*, the endophenotypes identified in the RDoC project may be the most useful groupings. But *for clinical* use, it is perfectly conceivable that, in the psychiatry of the future, we will conclude that many of the current diagnostic categories, for all their causal messiness, will prove to be the most practical ways to divide and classify the world of psychopathology. In the latter vein, Kendler and First argue that psychiatric nosology is not ready for a paradigm shift and that for now we should stick with improving the current categories in a progressive, iterative manner [31].

The final conclusion is that we may have to finally put the Robins/Guze validators to rest. We might achieve them with some narrowly defined endophenotypes as in the RDoC project, but it is unlikely that we will ever meet those standards with the larger diagnostic constructs needed for clinical practice. And with the demise of Robins/Guze we will need a new understanding of validity than the one associated with Robins/Guze criteria—a more flexible notion of validity that might change with the task to be accomplished.

References

1. Pouncey C. Mental disorders, like diseases, are constructs. So what? In: Phillips J, Frances A, et al. The six most essential questions in psychiatric diagnosis: a pluralogue. Part 1: conceptual and definitional issues in psychiatric diagnosis. Philos Ethics Humanit Med. 2012;7(3):1–29.
2. Robins E, Guze SB (1970) Establishment of diagnostic validity in psychiatric illness: its application to schizophrenia. Am J Psychiatry 126(7):983–7
3. Feighner JP, Robins E, Guze SB, Woodruff RA, Winokur G, Munoz R (1972) Diagnostic criteria for use in psychiatric research. Arch Gen Psychiatry 26:57–63
4. Spitzer RL, Endicott J, Robins E (1978) Research diagnostic criteria: rationale and reliability. Arch Gen Psychiatry 35:773–82
5. Regier DA, Narrow WE, Kuhl EA, Kupfer DJ (2009) The conceptual development of DSM-V. Am J Psychiatry 166(6):645–50
6. Kendler K (1990) Toward a scientific psychiatric nosology: strengths and limitations. Arch Gen Psychiatry 47:969–73
7. Hyman SE (2011) Diagnosis of mental disorders in light of modern genetics. In: Regier DA, Narrow WE, Kuhl EA, Kupfer DJ (eds) The conceptual evolution of DSM-5. American Psychiatric Publishing, Washington, DC, pp 3–18
8. Kupfer DJ, First MB, Regier DA (eds) (2002) A research agenda for DSM-V. American Psychiatric Association Press, Washington, DC
9. Craddock N, O'Donovan M, Owen M (2005) The genetics of schizophrenia and bipolar disorder: dissecting psychosis. J Med Genet 42:193–204
10. Craddock N, O'Donovan M, Owen M (2006) Genes for schizophrenia and bipolar disorder? Implications for psychiatric nosology. Schizophr Bull 32:9–16
11. Hyman SE (2008) A glimmer of light for neuropsychiatric disorders. Nature 455(16):890–3
12. Boyd J, Bur J, Gruenberg E, Holzer C et al (1984) Exclusion criteria of DSM-III: a study of co-occurrence of hierarchy-free syndromes. Arch Gen Psychiatry 41:983–9
13. Regier DA, Farmer M, Rae D, Locke B et al (1990) Comorbidity of mental disorders with alcohol and other drug abuse: results from the Epidemiologic Catchment Area (ECQ) study. J Am Med Assoc 26:2511–8
14. Kendell R, Jablensky A (2003) Distinguishing between the validity and utility of psychiatric diagnoses. Am J Psychiatry 160:4–12
15. Berrettini W (2000) Are schizophrenic and bipolar disorders related? A review of family and molecular studies. Biol Psychiatry 48:531–8
16. Lichtenstein P, Yip B, Bjork C et al (2009) Common genetic determinants of schizophrenia and bipolar disorder is Swedish families: a population-based study. Lancet 373:17–23
17. Kendler K (2006) Reflections on the relationship between psychiatric genetics and psychiatric nosology. Am J Psychiatry 163:1138–46

18. Phillips J. Symposium on DSM-5 (Part 1). Bulletin of the Association for the Advancement of Philosophy and Psychiatry. 2010;17(1):1–26. http://alien.dowling.edu/~cperring/aapp/bulletin.htm
19. Phillips J. Symposium on DSM-5 (Part 2). Association for the Advancement of Philosophy and Psychiatry. 2010;17(2):1–75. http://alien.dowling.edu/~cperring/aapp/bulletin.htm
20. Phillips J, Frances A et al (2012) The six most essential questions in psychiatric diagnosis: a pluralogue. Part 1: conceptual and definitional issues in psychiatric diagnosis. Philos Ethics Humanit Med 7(3):1–29
21. Kupfer DJ, Regier DA (2011) Neuroscience, clinical evidence, and the future of psychiatric classification in DSM-5. Am J Psychiatry 168(7):1–3
22. Hacking I (1999) The social construction of what? Harvard University Press, Cambridge, MA
23. Dupré J (1993) The disorder of things. Metaphysical foundations of the disunity of science. Harvard University Press, Cambridge, MA
24. Jablensky A (2012) The disease entity in psychiatry: fact or fiction. Epidemiol Psychiatr Sci 21:255–64
25. Kendler KS (2009) An historical frameword for psychiatric nosology. Psychol Med 39:1935–41
26. Bechtel W, Richardson RC (2010) Discovering complexity. Decomposition and localization as strategies in scientific research. MIT Press, Cambridge, MA
27. Kendler K (2005) "A Gene for…": the nature of gene action in psychiatric disorders. Am J Psychiatry 162:1243–52
28. Kendler K, Gardner C, Prescott C (2002) Toward a comprehensive developmental model for major depression in women. Am J Psychiatry 159:1133–45
29. Kendler K, Gardner C, Prescott C (2006) Toward a comprehensive developmental model for major depression in men. Am J Psychiatry 163:115–24
30. Kendler K (2012) The dappled nature of causes of psychiatric illness: replacing the organic-functional/hardware-software dichotomy with empirically based pluralism. Mol Biol 17:377–88
31. Kendler KS, First MB (2010) Alternative futures for the DSM revision process: iteration v. paradigm shift. Br J Psychiatry 197:263–5
32. Zachar P (2002) The practical kinds model as a pragmatist theory of classification. Philos Psychiatry Psychol 9:219–27

Chapter 11
Conclusion

James Phillips

Historical/Ideological Perspectives

DSM-5, along with its predecessors, claims to be no more nor less than a classification of psychiatric disorders. Each DSM aspires to carry out this classification mission in a scientific manner, organizing the world of psychopathology in the most scientifically acceptable manner at the time of its inscription. The authors of the successive manuals would thus be reluctant to see their creations as historical, cultural, ideological products rather than as scientific documents. The chapters in this section challenge the stated goals of the manuals by embedding the DSMs in their political contexts. In these other settings, the manuals become more and less than simple scientific nosologies: more in the sense that they are expressive of larger cultural themes; less in the sense that their science is inevitably thrown into question.

When the DSMs are viewed through the lenses of historical, cultural, political, and ideological contexts, what is revealed may be highly varied, depending on the particular lens and the particular interpreter. We begin with the dramatically different perspectives of Edward Shorter and John Sadler, the first with a micro-focus on the quirky roles of individuals in determining what will be the science of psychiatric nosology, the second with a macro-focus on the place of the DSMs in the vast world of the Mental Health Medical Industrial Complex (MHMIC). Joel Paris concludes this section with the biomedical ideology that is implicit in the two previous chapters.

J. Phillips (✉)
Department of Psychiatry, Yale School of Medicine,
88 Noble Avenue, New Haven, CT 06460, USA
e-mail: james.phillips@yale.edu

J. Paris and J. Phillips (eds.), *Making the DSM-5: Concepts and Controversies*,
DOI 10.1007/978-1-4614-6504-1_11, © Springer Science+Business Media New York 2013

Edward Shorter

Edward Shorter, prominent historian of psychiatry, provides us with a history of the DSMs, but it is not exactly a Whiggish account of ongoing progress toward an ever more scientific nosology. He gives us fair warning at the beginning of his chapter:

> Psychiatric diagnosis turns out to be complicated, probably far more so than anyone thought fifty years ago in the heyday of psychoanalysis when diagnoses didn't really count. And the story of the Diagnostic and Statistical Manual of the American Psychiatric Association is, at one level, a tale of steady progress in getting things right. At another level, it is the story of a nosological process that has, to some extent, run off the rails. Despite enormous investments of time, thought and academic firepower, the means of establishing a reliable nosology of psychiatric illness continues to slip from our grasp.

Shorter suggests that there are three approaches to creating a nolosogy: "reliance on authority, on consensus, or, the third, by identifying a disease by the 'medical model', a well-defined process that depends on more than 'consensus' in opinion or symptoms alone." In his account of the history of psychiatric nosology he details the extent to which the first two approaches have predominated over the third in major decisions. In the modern—supposedly more scientific—era, Emil Kraepelin loomed large as the decision maker. Shorter points to the complexity of this figure, on the one hand sensibly describing the goal of a nosology to "create small, homogeneous groups of patients whose illnesses had 'the same etiology, course, duration, and outcome'," and at the same time to erect "a firewall between the psychosis of dementia praecox and the affective troubles of manic-depressive illness."

With Kraepelin always in the background as an authority figure who wouldn't quite go away, Shorter moves on to the role of subsequent authorities and their effect on later nosologies. One such authority was William Menninger, whose World War II document, called Technical Medical Bulletin no. 203, was the predecessor of DSM-I and DSM-II. "The DSM series began with a document in the tradition of authoritarian pronunciamentos rather than consensus." Menninger's psychoanalytic bias indeed became a consensus of psychoanalytically oriented psychiatrists in the formation of the first two DSMs.

The conflict between authority and consensus then became quite dramatic in the 1970s, when psychopharmacologic agents and biology began to replace psychoanalysis as the new direction of psychiatry, and work was under way to develop DSM-III. The authority in question was Robert Spitzer, and the competing consensuses were the converging groups of biological psychiatrists from Washington University and Psychiatric Institute in New York, on the one hand, and the psychoanalytic association, on the other. As Shorter describes the process of developing the nosology, "…once the disease-designers were at the negotiating table, their approach more resembled horse-trading than admiration for science." Such horse-trading took place among the biological psychiatrists themselves, as well as between the biologists and the psychoanalysts. Spitzer's concession to the psychoanalysts to retain the word "neurosis" in DSM-III drew these responses from Donald Klein: "I must admit I was flabbergasted by this memo…Your current stand is, as far as I can see, entirely your own creation and was taken without either consultation with the Task Force or its agreement." And: "[Spitzer's insertion of neurosis] is clearly a response to political pressure, rather than a conceptual advance...To respond to this sort of unscientific and illogical, but sociologically understandable, pressure in the fashion that Dr. Spitzer suggests is unworthy of scientists who are attempting to advance our field via clarification and reliable definition."

In summing up the construction of DSM-III, Shorter points out that the new manual represented the victory of the Washington University biomedical model over psychoanalysis, but he underlines the triumph of authority over consensus.

> And here is the problem as we try to assess the DSM series within the force field of eminent-authority vs. committee-consensus nosology. On the face of it, the committee ruled, and the DSM-III drafters held many votes about which scientific issue was correct. Yet above these squabbling committees and their compromises lurked Spitzer—if the metaphor is pardonable—as a kind of master puppeteer, who invariably arranged for the outcome that he personally wished.

In moving onto DSM-IV Shorter emphasizes the conservative approach of Allen Frances in chairing the construction of that manual, and he concludes with the frustrated dreams of the DSM-5 Task Force to move beyond authority and consensus to a biomedical model. He concludes that "[t]he DSM is more a cultural than a scientific document." That statement leads us into John Sadler's chapter.

John Sadler

If Shorter hones down on a fine-grained analysis of the role of individual, authoritative, decisions in the construction of psychiatric nosologies, John Sadler moves in the opposite direction, approaching the DSMs from a highly macro perspective. In this analysis he actually diminishes the role of the DSM as the predominant force in American psychiatry by presenting it as one element (albeit an important one) in a much larger political-cultural phenomenon—what he calls the Mental Health Medical Industrial Complex (MHMIC).

Sadler introduces his chapter by noting the dominance of the DSM in American (and international) psychiatry since the publication of DSM-III in 1980. He questions how we are to explain the DSM hegemony. While acknowledging the scientific advances achieved by DSM-III and its successors, he discounts any explanation based simply on the manual's scientific merits. In seeking a more comprehensive explanation he begins with Dwight Eisenhower's famous, farewell warning about the dangers of a developing military industrial complex, and he quickly moves three decades forward to the application of Eisenhower's theme by Bernadine Healy, Chief of the National Institute of Mental Health from 1991 to 2003:

> If only we had remembered Eisenhower's less famous second warning: that 'public policy could itself become the captive of a scientific-technological elite' in which the 'power of money is ever present.' He feared elites would dominate the nation's scholars by virtue of their federal employment or their control over large research grants. Eisenhower was thinking about the solitary tinkerer overrun by task forces of scientists, but his instincts were prescient.

Sadler echoes Healy's concern that an analogous medical industrial complex has developed, which he names the Mental Health Medical Industrial Complex (MHMIC), and he offers a straightforward statement of his thesis about the DSM: "Regarding the dominance of the DSM, my thesis is simple. The DSM has prevailed because it has, on balance, served its function in the MHMIC, whose monolithic influences on funding, public policy, and the social discourse on mental illness reinforces the DSM's stability and success." He adds that DSM's role in the MHMIC dictates a conservative attitude toward change, since the MHMIC is already in place, and its faithful lieutenant, DSM, has its designated place in the larger regiment. Since, for Sadler, to understand the DSM we have to understand the MHMIC, he proceeds to an analysis of the latter.

Sadler breaks the MHMIC into ten elements, all "'conspir[ing]' to stabilize a DSM with minimal changes." Element 1 is *Millions of mentally ill people*, a target group available for potential exploitation, and requiring classification by the DSM. Element 2 is the *Pharmaceutical industry*. The ever expanding list of DSM psychiatric disorders provides new indications for pharmaceutical intervention. The tendency of the DSMs to overlap with and medicalize ordinary life suffering provides further opportunities for Pharma. And the tendency of DSM categories to overlap, with increasing comorbidities, converges with the cross-indications and off-label use of pharmaceutical agents.

Element 3 is the *For-profit service industry*. The health insurance increases profit by reducing care. The DSM plays its role in this maneuver by providing diagnoses that lend themselves to cheap drug therapy as opposed to more drawn-out, expensive psychosocial interventions. Further, drug trials are easier to carry out on DSM categories than evaluations of psychosocial interventions. Element 4 is the *US healthcare system*. Traditional American individualism has interacted with major lobbying efforts to prevent universal health care. Support for the existing healthcare structure militates against any real change in our diagnostic system.

Element 5 is *US Politics*. Corporate, insurance, and pharmaceutical interests play a huge role, including the expenditure of massive amounts of lobbying expenditures, to keep the MHMIC in place. That includes keeping the DSM in its place in the MHMIC. Element 6 is *Advertising and mass media*. This category reflects another aspect of the phenomenon discussed under Element 5, the application of massive financial resources to maintain the status quo.

Element 7 is the *NIMH*. Sadler reviews the very interesting history of the NIMH, initiated in 1949 and funded by Congress to develop research programs into the causes and treatment of mental illness. Under its first leader, Robert Felix, the NIMH was active in developing community alternatives to state hospitals. In latter decades the agency has turned its focus onto neuroscience and biomedical treatments. Sadler reflects on the relationship that has developed between the NIMH and the pharmaceutical industry.

The *de facto* arrangement of taxpayer-supported basic science through NIH, with clinical trials referred to the pharmaceutical industry for sponsorship, amounts to a taxpayer subsidy of the pharmaceutical industry's research and development. The NIMH does the basic and translational science, whose results in the public sphere can be appropriated by the pharmaceutical companies in the development of new therapeutic agents. In the meantime, fundamental and important questions regarding health services, psychosocial treatments, conceptual issues, public health, and patient initiatives remain marginally unfunded. One final note is that NIMH funded research projects are reviewed by leaders in the field whose careers have been made in research based on DSM categories. There is thus little incentive to break the DSM lock on research. Sadler points out later in the chapter that the NIMH RDoC project may represent a significant departure from that trend.

Element 8 is *Popular demand*. Popular demand for non-pharmacologic, non-DSM-based treatments has no support in the DSM or pharmacological communities, nor, more generally, in the MHMIC. Element 9 is *Academic medical centers*. Over recent decades research has shifted from the individual "physician-scientist" to the academic medical centers (AMCs), and the latter have assumed their role as one more cog in the MHMIC, depending highly on support from the NIMH and big Pharma, with all the challenges to integrity involved in those relationships.

Element 10, last but certainly not least, is the *American Psychiatric Association*. The obvious point is the AMA's ownership of the DSM manuals and the tens of millions of dollars made from sale of the manuals. "The degree to which profitability determines DSM policy remains a secret of the APA leadership." The AMA's financial dependence on the DSM puts it inevitably in a compromised position: manual revisions frequently enough to maintain profit flow; enough changes in the revisions to give them credibility.

In his discussion and conclusion, Sadler cautions that his critique of the MHMIC, and the DSM as a major piece of that larger structure, should not be viewed as a demonizing of those entities. As he says, "I should acknowledge that the MHMIC provides the only credible resource for developing, testing, and promulgating products to help doctors help patients. What concerned Eisenhower and Bernadine Healy was the idea that the "moneyed elites" have profound potential to compromise other important values and missions for the country. Similarly, the moneyed elites have profound potential to corrupt other important values and missions for psychiatry, mental health and their affiliated institutions." Sadler proceeds at length to outline ways, big and small, in which the excesses of the MHMIC could be mitigated. He ends on a guardedly optimistic note:

> Regarding the DSM, many possibilities for change are possible. The DSM-5 Task Force promised a manual with big changes when in the early stages of work, but current trends seem to suggest backpedaling on innovations, perhaps in response to outcries of protest. Perhaps NIMH's interest in the RDoC idea signals a new responsiveness to other and more alternatives to the DSM. Perhaps the DSM-5 idea about a 'living document' may lead into support for 'open source' classifications of disorder, subject to testing and modification by anyone with a panel of patients who are interested. Only time will tell.

Joel Paris

Joel Paris' chapter, "The Ideology behind DSM-5," forms a perfect complement to the chapters of Shorter and Sadler, explicitly stating a theme that hovers in the background of their chapters. Paris' theme is that the DSMs, starting with DSM-III continuing with DSM-5, are driven by an ideology of the biomedical model—that mental disorders can be fully explained by neuroscience. This theme was present in Shorter's chapter, as he noted that while the stated aim of DSM-III was to be descriptive and atheoretical, the architects of the manual—both the St. Louis and New York groups—were strongly wedded to a biomedical position. Their goal, with Spitzer in the lead, was to dislodge psychoanalysis from its prominent place in DSM-II and replace it with a "neo-Kraepelian" manual.

In the case of Sadler's chapter, the biomedical model could have been included as an 11th element in the MHMIC. It is implicit, however, in several of the stated elements, most dramatically in Element 2 (pharmaceutical industry), Element 3 (for-profit service industry), Element 7 (NIMH), Element 8 (popular demand), and Element 9 (academic medical centers). Further, the diagram presents the ten elements as spokes around the biomedically oriented DSM hub. Sadler argues in several places that biomedical orientation of DSM and the MHMIC have pushed other psychosocial interventions off the playing field. Just as the economic motive weaves its way through Sadler's analysis, so also does the ideology of the biomedical model.

Paris begins his chapter with a statement of medical modesty:

Medicine is a practical discipline. A classification of disease is primarily intended for communication, and is usually provisional. The mechanisms of only a few diseases are understood well enough for diagnosis to be firmly based on science. Diagnostic systems are particularly bound to be messy in psychiatry, a field that concerns the vast complexities of mind and brain.

He then explains how advances in the various tools of neuroscience have created the illusion that these findings will lead to a definitive explanation of mental disorders. He regrets the loss of a richer biopsychosocial model, and he cites a recent statement by the editors of DSM-5 that the ever-desired, ever-elusive paradigm shift for the post-DSM-5 manuals will come from the neuroscientific research of the NIMH RDoC project [1]. Given the fact that this research is in its infancy, with minimal conclusive findings, and still not a single biomarker for any major DSM category, the confidence expressed that the important answers will all come from the RDoC and other neuroscientific research has to be called an ideology. "Given the limited state of evidence in support of [RDoC] spectra, the adoption of RDoCs by NIMH can only be described as ideological."

In trying to explain psychiatry and DSM's embrace of the ideology of neuroscience, Paris points to the field's "internist envy," the wish to attain the respectability of other medical specialties, both by other physicians and by the general public. It is difficult to accept the fact that, due to the complexity of the brain, psychiatry remains at the syndromal stage where other specialties were almost a century ago. We are left with the alternatives of urging neuroscience to push us rapidly forward, or to come to terms with the fact that psychiatry is indeed not just another biomedical specialty.

Ideological *and* Conceptual Perspectives

The second three chapters in the volume continue the themes of historical and ideological analysis, but now with more of an emphasis on conceptual analysis regarding the nature of psychiatric disorders. The first three chapters did of course include conceptual analysis in their enquiries into history and ideology. The next three chapters simply shift the balance more in the direction of conceptual analysis.

Warren Kinghorn

The title of Warren Kinghorn's chapter, "The Biopolitics of Defining 'Mental Disorder,'" alerts us that we haven't left history and politics behind. Kinghorn begins with psychiatry's struggle to define itself. The definition to which the profession is reduced, that psychiatry is the specialty that treats mental disorders, leads immediately to the need to define "mental disorder," and that in turn leads to circular definitions, as well as to the anti-psychiatry critique that psychiatry constructs mental disorders to create a justification for the work. Kinghorn alerts us early on that he will not provide the desired definition, and further that he will argue that the search for definition has little to do with the scientific need for said definition and much to do with the political search for a "safe place" for the practice of psychiatry.

In exploring this issue Kinghorn takes us back to the 1970s, effectively picking up the conversation with Edward Shorter. With DSM-I and II, there was apparently no felt need to provide a definition of mental disorder, and none was provided in either manual. But the 1970s witnessed the anti-psychiatry attacks on psychiatry's legitimacy, and in addition the profession was shaken by the embarrassing episode in which the disease status of homosexuality was decided by a membership vote. In the face of these troubles leaders in the field felt a need to shore up the legitimacy of the profession by developing a clear understanding and definition of mental disorder. The challenge to accomplish this mission fell to—you guessed it—Robert Spitzer, chair of the APA Task Force on Nomenclature and Statistics and then, as we have heard from Shorter, main architect of DSM-III. Along the way Spitzer had also negotiated the compromise solution over homosexuality, and was especially sensitive to psychiatry's need to define itself. Quoting Kinghorn, "Spitzer and Jean Endicott stated that the homosexuality controversy provided the 'initial impetus' for the effort to place a definition of mental disorder in DSM-III…They stated that the conviction that a definition was needed grew as the DSM-III revision process began in 1975…'Decisions had to be made on a variety of issues that seemed to relate to the fundamental question of the boundaries of the concept of mental disorder. We believed that without some definition of mental disorder, there would be no explicit guiding principles that would help to determine which conditions should be included in the nomenclature, which excluded, and how included conditions should be defined.'"

The decision to formulate a definition of mental disorder for DSM-III was only the beginning of the struggle to actually agree on a definition. Spitzer's proposal to define mental disorder as a subset of medical disorder was met with opposition, especially by the American Psychological Association, and he finally agreed on a compromise, watered-down definition, with the qualifier that "there is no satisfactory definition that specifies precise boundaries for the concept 'mental disorder'"—in this case, then, in Shorter's terms, the authority submitting to the pressure of the consensus.

DSM-III thus provided the first official definition of mental disorder, albeit with the irony that the biomedically oriented manual was not allowed to use the word "medical" in the definition. As Kinghorn notes, the DSM-III definition has remained the basis for the definitions in all subsequent manuals, including, presumably, DSM-5.

Kinghorn argues convincingly that despite intentions that a formal definition of mental disorder should play a substantive role in functional questions such as whether to allow a new diagnostic category into the manual, the definition has never—in DSM-III or in any of it successors—played such a role. Rather, it tends to get tacked onto the respective manual after the real work has been accomplished. Why then, Kinghorn asks, is it there? Does it serve any purpose at all? He writes:

> I suggest here that the DSM-5 definition of mental disorder, like its predecessors in DSM-III, DSM-III-R, and DSM-IV, serves a function which is primarily political. To the extent that the definition exerts influence, I argue, it does so by constructing the way that psychiatry is interpreted as a medical specialty—both by psychiatrists themselves and by the larger communities within which psychiatry is practiced—and consequently by constructing the way that individuals in our culture grant authority to psychiatry and psychiatry's diagnostic language.

Kinghorn goes on to say that, as opposed to providing a regulative function in the admission of diagnoses, or a philosophical account of the nature of mental disorder, what the definition accomplishes is to "delineate the rough boundaries of a clinical 'space' within which psychiatry as a medical discipline exercises proper authority and which does not encroach on territory which is socially and politically controversial."

In delineating how the definitions go about securing the clinical space within which psychiatry can comfortably work, Kinghorn describes three ways in which the definitions accomplish their goal, one of which is subtle and very interesting. All the definitions of mental disorder employ special images of depth and interiority to "affirm that mental disorders are interior to individuals and that they somehow underlie the distress, disability, and impairment of function which is associated with them." Kinghorn notes that the definitions of mental disorder place the dysfunction *in* the patient, as opposed to speaking of dysfunctions *of* the patient, as with nonpsychiatric illnesses. In this subtle linguistic distinction between the use of "in" and "of," psychiatry has carved out a "safe place" for its unique work.

Following this careful linguistic analysis, Kinghorn goes on to argue that in fact it doesn't work. "Far from defending psychiatry against anti-psychiatric critique, the DSM definitions in fact display the high degree to which psychiatric diagnosis is both value-laden and politically contestable." He provides three reasons for this conclusion. The first is that for most psychiatric diagnoses you can't demonstrate a dysfunction *in* the patient that causes the dysfunction *of* the patient. The second is that the concept of "function," as in dysfunction, remains a socially contestable concept. Who can judge what is normal functioning and what is dysfunction? "Here again, the DSM definitions of mental disorder do not rescue psychiatric diagnosis from sociopolitical critique and controversy: rather, in invoking the concept of function, they display the degree to which psychiatric diagnosis depends on normative standards which are themselves socially contestable." Finally, the third reason why the DSM definitions fail psychiatry is that the location of dysfunction *in* the individual involves psychiatry in the entire history of modern Western individualism and in that way provincializes psychiatry into a Western medical enterprise.

Kinghorn ends with the dramatic conclusion that we abandon efforts to define our specialty, remove the definition from DSM-5, and accept the challenge of doing our work without the desired foundational definition. "A psychiatry willing to go on without a definition of mental disorder would be a psychiatry without foundations— but since the present foundations cannot hold the weight place upon them, that is just where psychiatry needs to be."

Douglas Porter

Douglas Porter's chapter, Establishing Normative Validity for Scientific Psychiatric Nosology: The Significance of Integrating Patient Perspectives, readily connects to the two chapters that precede it. On the one hand, Porter's emphasis on the normative dimension of psychiatric diagnosis can be readily related to Kinghorn's work on definition. In his analysis of psychiatric efforts to develop a definition of mental disorder, Kinghorn noted that the definitions got hung up on normative dimensions of the concept of dysfunction. A biomedical definition of mental disorder that builds "dysfunction" into the definition simply self-destructs. On the other hand, Porter's focus on the implicit evaluative dimension of Kraepelinian and neo-Kraepelinian empiricism is a restatement in other language of Paris' analysis of the ideology of the biomedical model. A further point in making these connections is that, regarding Kinghorn's conclusion that psychiatry has failed in its effort to establish a foundation for the specialty, Porter might respond that it is biomedical psychiatry that has failed in establishing a foundation for *its* psychiatry, and that the question of foundation remains open in the broader conception of psychiatry proposed by Porter.

Porter begins the chapter with a review of the supposedly atheoretical view of the neo-Kraepelinian, biomedical model developed by the St. Louis school, that received its most articulate and influential expression by Robins and Guze in their classic article in 1970 [2]. In the use of this model for the development of DSM-III, all involved assumed that the psychoanalytically biased DSM-II was to be replaced with a "descriptive" atheoretical approach—that the biomedical model was not itself one more ideology. Porter quotes the self-contradicting statement of Comptom and Guze that "[t]he medical model is without a priori theory, but does consider brain mechanisms to be a priority" [3]. He relates the expectation of the architects of DSM-III that the diagnostic categories that achieved reliability in that manual would with further research meet the Robins/Guze standards of validity.

What followed is well known: further research did not achieve the desired Robins/Guze validity for DSM diagnoses. Porter notes that this failure at validation has not deterred the Task Force of DSM-5 from asserting its biomedical goal: it has simply not been accomplished yet. In the meantime psychosocial aspects of mental disorders have been mostly ignored in the search for biomedical validation.

Porter now turns back to Karl Jaspers, who was already arguing in 1913 that psychological presentations of psychiatric disorders would probably not neatly map onto neuroscientific substrates. He proposed an ideal-type organization of psychiatric presentations, arguing that such grouping could lead to productive intervention, even in the absence of formal disease status for the respective diagnostic categories. Porter moves into the present by citing the work of Kenneth Kendler, who has demonstrated complex, interacting factors—psychological, social, etc.—that play roles along with biological factors in the development of psychopathology.

For Porter the recognition of a pluralistic approach to etiology and nosology leads us toward an appreciation of the normative dimension of nosology. He invokes the work of the sociologist/philosopher Jürgen Habermas to assert that the recognition of values in the construction of a nosology does not mean a loss of objectivity for a relativistic, anything-goes free-for-all. The fact is that there are always values: the effort to hew to a rigidly biomedical model is itself a value, as shown by Paris in the previous chapter.

Porter concludes by arguing that a full, value-respectful nosology will make a place for patients in the nosology. "While patients are the preeminent stakeholders in terms of the institutional impact of nosology they have traditionally been the most marginalized in terms of impact upon development of nosology. Normative validity entails a more significant role for patients in the development of nosology." Porter closes with an interesting and appropriate debate between Flanagan, Davidson, and Strauss, on the one hand, and Cuthbert and Insel on the other, regarding the respective usefulness of first-person accounts vs. neuro-circuitry, RDoC data in the understanding of schizophrenia [4–6].

Owen Whooley and Allan V. Horwitz

In The Paradox of Professional Success: Grand Ambition, Furious Resistance, and the Derailment of the DSM-Revision Process, Owen Whooley and Allan Horwitz pick up some of the themes from other chapters and develop them from the perspective of dimensional measures in DSM-5. They organize their chapter around one signal event. During the week of May 8, 2012, in the context of the annual meeting of the American Psychiatric Association in Philadelphia, the APA Assembly voted unanimously to relegate the proposed dimensional scales in DSM-5 to an appendix of the manual for further study. The Assembly cited the "undue burden" that the "unproven severity scales" would place on clinicians. The Assembly vote, followed by an editorial in the New York Times by Allen Frances criticizing the entire DSM-5 process, stirred a degree of attention one would not expect from a decision about a diagnostic manual. This chapter is devoted to explaining the significance of that vote.

Whooley and Horwitz begin by taking us back to the era we have visited in other chapters, the psychiatric tumult of the 1970s, culminating in the publication of DSM-III in 1980. They review the effort to legitimize the profession of psychiatry as a medical specialty through the biomedically oriented DSM-III. Once again placing Robert Spitzer in his pivotal role, they write: "In 1980, Robert Spitzer essentially transformed what was a document largely incidental to professional practice into the final word on defining both the universe of mental disorders and the identity of psychiatry itself." The effort was successful, and psychiatry enjoyed a period of newly found prestige, a prestige that was strongly identified with the status achieved by DSM-III.

In the ensuing years, however, the flaws in DSM-III began to emerge and create a new crisis of legitimacy. In the terminology with which we are now familiar, DSM-III achieved reliability and promised that validity would follow with further research. In 1994 DSM-IV was published in an attitude of caution and conservatism. Since science had not yet provided validation for the diagnostic categories, the better wisdom was to keep changes minimal in the expectation of further scientific advance. As we know, the 1990s, the decade of the brain, again failed to produce the desired validation. The diagnostic categories continued to stick out like houses built on sand. The architects of DSM-5 saw it as their challenge to produce a corrective document. The prestige of the DSM—and of the APA—was on the line. They began in the early years of the new century with a promise and expectation that the neuroscience would be in place to shore up the diagnostic categories. It quickly became clear that not only would neuroscience and genetics not be ready to validate the DSM categories in time for DSM-5 (originally scheduled for 2010, now moved to May, 2013), they would in fact probably never be ready. What we have in fact learned from neuroscience and genetics is that the diagnostic categories do not represent genuine phenotypes that will match up with straightforward genotypes and neuroscientific irregularities.

The DSM-5 response to this crisis of unfilled validation was to move toward a dimensional conceptualization of mental disorders. Whooley and Horwitz provide a detailed description of the proposed dimensional measures, cross-cutting measures to be used with all patients and severity measures for particular diagnoses. They explain the implications for a nosology of taking a dimensional rather than categorical approach to mental disorders. They explain the growing discord in the profession regarding the switch to dimensions. In the beginning the debate was carried out among the "experts," but eventually moved to the rank and file. From a technical perspective the dimensional measures were criticized as unproven and untested. From a practical perspective the measures were constructed in a way that, completely aside from their questionable value, would take excessive amounts of time to administer, almost guaranteeing their not being used in clinical practice. In that context the APA Assembly took the dramatic step of removing the measures from the front of the new manual.

The authors conclude with a reflection on the excessive burden placed on the DSM to accomplish conflicting tasks, in addition to carrying the prestige of the APA. They conclude: "Psychiatry's persistent, vexing problem is that its excessive expectations of the DSM are a guarantee that the DSM will not be able to fulfill any of them adequately."

Conceptual Perspectives

The final chapters of the volume leave political and ideological issues behind and focus on purely conceptual factors. There's no better place to start than with Allen Frances' reflections. He brings to the discussion his experience as Chair of the DSM-IV Task Force, and in that way fills in some of the discussion of earlier chapters on the history of the DSMs. He has of course achieved new prominence as a critic of the DSM-5 process. That is reflected in this chapter, but of more significance is his discussion of conceptual problems that existed in DSM-IV and remain operative in DSM-5. In the next chapter Joseph Pierre analyzes the conflict over setting diagnostic thresholds and the effort to balance sensitivity and specificity, or false positives and false negatives. Aaron Mishara and Michael Schwartz follow with a chapter arguing for the merits (and lack of presence) of the phenomenological perspective in the DSMs. In the final chapter James Phillips addresses the question of how psychiatric nosology might look in the future.

Allen Frances

Allen Frances covers three areas in his chapter: epistemological/ontological status of psychiatric disorders; definition of psychiatric disorder; and conservative vs. aggressive approaches toward changes in DSM-5. In the first section he invokes a baseball metaphor of three umpires: the first representing a realist approach to the status of psychiatric diagnoses, the second a hybrid realist/constructivist approach, and the third a purely constructivist approach. He invokes Robert Spitzer to represent the first umpire, Thomas Szasz to represent the third umpire, and himself as the second umpire. His second-umpire position ("There are balls and there are strikes and I call them as I see them") is that psychiatric illness exists in the real world, and that our diagnostic constructs are our fallible efforts to reflect the illnesses we deal with. The fact that the diagnoses are constructs—some more accurate, some less accurate—does not mean that we are inventing illnesses, only that our effort to capture them accurately with our diagnostic categories is open to error. He rejects the first-umpire position that our diagnostic categories map neatly onto the field of real-world psychopathology, as well as the third-umpire position that psychiatric disorders are nothing other than social constructs of our making.

He questions why progress in psychiatric science has not been as smooth as that in other sciences:

Descriptive classification in psychiatry has so far been singularly unsuccessful in promoting a breakthrough discovery of the causes of mental disorder. This is doubly disappointing given the miraculous advances in our understanding of normal brain functioning. The advances in molecular biology, brain imaging, and genetics are spectacular—their impact on understanding psychopathology almost nil. Why the disconnect?

His response to his question is the complexity of psychiatric disorders. In other terminology, our current diagnostic categories may not represent real phenotypes that will lend themselves to normal scientific analysis.

In the second section of the chapter Frances takes up the question of definition of mental disorder. In discussing definition he is in partial agreement with Kinghorn's analysis and in partial disagreement. He is in agreement that numerous efforts to define mental illness (including the one in which he participated in DSM-IV) have largely failed. He adds that "[t]his is a hole at the center of psychiatric classification." Where he disagrees with Kinghorn is around the question of what to do about it. While Kinghorn favors giving up the effort and removing from the DSM a definition that doesn't work and that we don't need anyway, Frances (in a dialogue with Kinghorn published elsewhere) argues that, imperfect as it is, the definition serves a purpose and should be retained [7].

In a final section Frances argues strongly for a conservative approach in making changes in DSM-5. His first argument is that, inasmuch as the DSM-III diagnostic categories have still not been validated scientifically, change should only follow demonstrated validity for a respective change. In the face of missing validity, we should emphasize clarity of description and practical utility:

On the other hand, if you believe as I do, that the DSM is necessarily more an exercise in forging a common language than in finding a truth, you need a strong reason to change the syntax. And it turns out that such strong evidence is usually lacking. This is why the reliability and utility goals are so important (and for all the discussion about it, validation is not yet particularly meaningful).

Frances' second argument for a conservative approach is the potential for unforeseen, real-world consequences of making even minor changes in the existing manual. As examples of this phenomenon in the conservative DSM-IV manual, he mentions the misuse of the Paraphilia NOS category to justify the extended civil commitment of sexual offenders who have reached the end of their sentences, and the unexpected diagnostic inflation of bipolar diagnoses, and attendant use of mood-stabilizing and neuroleptic medications, that followed the introduction of the Bipolar II category into DSM-IV.

Joseph Pierre

In Overdiagnosis, Underdiagnosis, Synthesis: A Dialectic for Psychiatry and the DSM, Joseph Pierre takes up a topic addressed by Allen Frances in his discussion of diagnostic and criterial expansion. Frances' concern was centered on overtreatment, the incidence of creating a population of false positives with new diagnoses and lowered thresholds. Pierre attempts to examine this issue in an intensive, nuanced, and balanced manner. He begins by addressing the fact that, in the absence of bio-markers and other validity measures with psychiatric diagnoses, we are unavoidably caught in a struggle to decide on appropriate thresholds in framing our criteria for presence or absence of a particular diagnosis. In the first part of his chapter he reviews the concerns about excessive sensitivity—allowing for overdiagnosis and false positives in order to assure the treatment of afflicted individuals—and the concerns about excessive specificity—allowing for undertreatment and false negatives in order to avoid treating unafflicted individuals.

Regarding the first, he points to tendencies in both the psychoanalytically oriented pre-DSM-III era and the post-DSM-III biomedical era toward an overin-clusion of individuals in the respective diagnostic categories. This involves both an encroachment on the boundaries of normal and an overuse of psychiatric medica-tions for increasingly questionable indications. Regarding the concerns over under-treatment and false negatives, Pierre reviews findings such as the undertreatment of depression in primary care, as well as the neglect of those with mild and subthresh-old symptoms.

In trying to find a balance between over- and undertreatment, Pierre makes a number of points. The first is that increasing the number of diagnoses does not nec-essarily mean diagnostic creep; it may mean nothing more than splitting the existing diagnoses into subgroups. A second point is that, in the absence of clear biological markers, the issue of "clinically significant distress" and diagnostic threshold will always involve subjective judgment. A related phenomenon is that both epidemio-logic surveys carried out by lay interviewers and evaluations by involved clinicians tend to use low thresholds in their estimations of who suffers from a mental disor-der. Regarding the latter Pierre writes: "clinicians considering whether an individual should be treated will tend to have a very low threshold to define caseness. The principle of inclusiveness that has focused on minimizing false negatives at the pos-sible expense of including false positives is therefore defensible on the grounds that DSM's 'highest priority has been to provide a helpful guide to clinical practice.'" Other situations that may alter how the threshold of clinical significance is set are public mental health settings with limited resources, forensic settings with their own priorities, and research settings with their priorities. In this mix of circumstances Pierre emphasizes clinical utility as the preeminent criterion that should determine where diagnostic thresholds are set.

Following a discussion of Attenuated Psychosis Syndrome as exemplary of the issues involved in setting diagnostic thresholds, Pierre concludes with a reflection on the future. In trying to find a balance between over- and underdiagnosis, he endorses the current direction of DSM-5 toward a dimensional view of psychiatric diagnosis. Against the critics' concern over overdiagnosis, Pierre makes a compari-son with general medicine:

> Over the course of our lives, having a transient or chronic physical illness and receiving medical treatment is completely normal and to be expected. Since its inception, general medical practice has managed suffering associated with pain, coughs, broken bones,

pregnancy, aging, and the process of dying independent of debate about whether these conditions represent "harmful dysfunctions." There is no *a priori* reason why that should differ for psychiatry.

Pierre notes further that, if mental health dysfunction is conceptualized on a continuum with normal, everyday functioning, that will involve a range of treaters, with psychiatrists with their medications filling a role at one end of the spectrum, as opposed to being the exclusive treaters of all conditions deemed mentally troubled.

> Expanding DSM's concept of mental disorder within a continuum model makes sense within the larger scope of public mental health care, but economic realities, risk-benefit analyses, and neuroethical concerns should limit parallel expansion of the scope of treatment by psychiatrists in kind. In this sense, DSM can sidestep the threshold problem by embracing a more continuous model of mental health-mental illness, but outside of the microcosm of private practice, debates about the proper thresholds to trigger specific intervention by psychiatrists will linger on.

Aaron Mishara and Michael Schwartz

In What does Phenomenology Contribute to the Debate about DSM-5, Aaron Mishara and Michael Schwartz argue that the tradition of philosophical phenomenology has a major contribution on offer to the DSMs that the latter have not taken advantage of. In introducing their theme they hasten to provide terminological clarifications regarding the words "phenomenology" and "subjectivity." In ordinary psychiatric usage "phenomenology" refers to the collection of symptoms in filling out diagnostic criteria, as well as to the related notion of describing the patient's individual, subjective experience. Mishara and Schwartz clarify that phenomenology in the tradition of philosopher Edmund Husserl refers rather to the use of individual, subjective experiences as a first step in the disciplined study of the structure of subjective experience. This is important, given the common use of "subjective" to mean only the individual, private, and personal. They fault Allen Frances for dismissing phenomenology because of his assumption of the latter misunderstanding. They also point out that DSM operational definitions don't even capture individual, subjective experience because the evaluation is so focused on checking off symptoms in the diagnostic criteria. Their main argument is that a disciplined analysis of subjective experience will reveal both the structure of ordinary experience and the deviations from that structure that constitute psychopathology—and that provide guidance for discovering correlations with neuroscientific findings.

At another level of analysis of subjective experience, the authors invoke the Husserlian analysis of perception in terms of typifications, the way in which ordinary perception involves the use of categories (e.g., I look at that tree, but I see it as a tree because I bring my category of tree to the experience). They argue that we follow a similar proceeding in our diagnostic evaluations. We use diagnostic typifications as we quickly (and even unconsciously) locate the patient in one of our diagnostic categories. The fact that the categories may not represent real phenotypes is not a problem, as they are only the starting point in diagnosis and are subject to ongoing revision and clarification.

Finally, the authors argue that a DSM with a more phenomenological orientation would be a manual without the current conflict between clinical and research interests. An emphasis on real subjective experience would satisfy clinical needs, and the focus on the structures of such experience would provide material for potential neuroscientific correlations.

James Phillips

As James Phillips relates in the final chapter, the DSM process achieved the triumph of the biomedical model with DSM-III in 1980. That landmark document introduced a symptom-based, descriptive approach to diagnosis, with operational definitions of the diagnostic categories accomplished through the use of diagnostic criteria. The manual achieved the desired goal of reliability in diagnosis across treatment and research settings. The architects of DSM-III assumed that diagnostic validity, using the Robins/Guze criteria published 10 years before DSM-III, would follow with the burgeoning science in the post-DSM-III era. As Phillips relates, the story of the ensuing decades has been that of validity failure, with the unavoidable conclusion that the diagnostic categories do not represent real phenotypes. This story then carries into the failed efforts of the DSM-5 authors to fill in the validity breach with a variety of measures, including reorganization of the diagnoses, introduction of new diagnoses, and primarily an effort to supplement the categorical approach of the previous DSMs with a variety of dimensional measures. With the failure of its innovations to accomplish very much, DSM-5 has cast its lot with the NIMH Research Domain Criteria (RDoC) project and the promise of that innovative approach to bring some degree of scientific validity to psychiatric nosology. In an effort to imagine what psychiatric nosology might look like in the post-DSM-5 era, Phillips applies the philosophy of science tools of natural kind analysis and complexity theory to psychiatric classification. The result is a view of psychiatric disorders as conditions with very complex etiologies, and with no one valid way in which the world of psychopathology should be sorted out and classified. This will lead to a notion of diagnostic validity quite different from that of Robins and Guze.

As should surprise no one, these chapters do not culminate in a grand conclusion about the DSMs. The manuals — and the opinions — are too complex for that kind of ending. The goal of this volume has rather been to open and promote discussion of the many issues and unanswered questions concerning the DSMs.

References

1. Kupfer DJ, Regier DA. Neuroscience, clinical evidence, and the future of psychiatric classification in DSM-5. Am J Psychiatry. 2011;168:172–4.
2. Robins E, Guze SB. Establishment of diagnostic validity in psychiatric illness: its application to schizophrenia. Am J Psychiatry. 1970;126:983–7.

3. Compton WM, Guze SB. The neo-Kraepelinian revolution in psychiatric diagnosis. Eur Arch Psychiatry Clin Neurosci. 1995;245:196–201.
4. Flanagan EH, Davidson L, Strauss JS. Issues for DSM-5: incorporating patients' subjective experiences. Am J Psychiatry. 2007;164:391–2.
5. Flanagan EH, Davidson L, Strauss JS. The need for patient-subjective data in the DSM and the ICD. Psychiatry. 2010;73:297–307.
6. Cuthbert B, Insel T. The data of diagnosis: new approaches to psychiatric classification. Psychiatry. 2010;73:311–4.
7. Phillips J, Frances A, et al. The six most essential questions in psychiatric diagnosis: a pluralogue. Part 1: conceptual and definitional issues in psychiatric diagnosis. Philos Ethics Humanit Med. 2012;7(3):1–29.

References

Index

J. Paris and J. Phillips (eds.), *Making the DSM-5: Concepts and Controversies,*
DOI 10.1007/978-1-4614-6504-1, © Springer Science+Business Media New York 2013